Enhancing Performance and Quality of Life Guide

Enhancing Performance and Quality of Life Guide

Steven J. Danish
Tanya Forneris

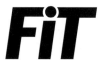

FiT Publishing
A Division of the International Center of
Performance Excellence
West Virginia University - CPASS
375 Birch Street
P.O. Box 6116
Morgantown, WV 26506-6116

Library of Congress Card Catalog Number: 2017956467

ISBN: 9781940067278

Cover Design: Wendy Lazzell, FiT Publishing
Cover Photos: iStock.com | Credit: fzant, Stock photo ID: 182025924
Ladder Photo: iStock.com | Credit: owattaphotos, Stock photo ID: 696322396
Typesetter: Wendy Lazzell, FiT Publishing
Production Editor: Eileen Harvey

10 9 8 7 6 5 4 3 2 1

FiT Publishing
A Division of the International Center for Performance Excellence
West Virginia University
375 Birch Street, WVU-CPASS
PO Box 6116
Morgantown, WV 26506-6116
800.477.4348 (toll free)
304.293.6888 (phone)
304.293.6658 (fax)
Email: fitcustomerservice@mail.wvu.edu
Website: www.fitpublishing.com

Table of Contents

Introduction

Our textbook, *Enhancing Performance and Quality of Life*, is designed to help professional groups that work with adults and youth how to teach life skills. However, we learned that many readers wanted to learn life skills on their own and be able to teach it to others, especially youth. For this reason we developed this *Guide*. Part I is written to be self-guided for adult readers to learn or review the life skills on their own and at their own pace. Part II is designed to help those working with youth, whether individually (e.g., parent, religious or secular mentor, or teacher) or in groups (e.g., coaches, youth program leaders, teachers), to foster the development of life skills for youth.

Many readers may already be familiar and have some experience with these life skills. However, because we believe in social action, we do not believe that simply learning the skills from a textbook format is sufficient. We have had many individuals tell us they wanted the opportunity to learn and review the skills on their own. In 1969, at his Presidential address to the American Psychological Association, George Miller talked about giving psychology away as a means of providing psychological knowledge and expertise to the public at little or no charge. This is our effort toward giving psychology away, or at least providing it at minimal cost. Another advantage of Part I of this guide is that such an approach need not be provided to the public only if they have problems requiring therapy. We all lack some of the skills to live successfully. Just as being a poor speller does not mean you have a spelling disorder, not knowing how to make effective decisions does not mean you have a decision-making disorder.

The rationale for including Part II of this guide is because it is also critical for youth to develop life skills in order to succeed in life. Youth are taking more risks with their health, their lives, and their future than ever before. Involvement in behaviors such as drug use, unprotected and unsafe sex, violent and delinquent acts, and dropping out of school continue to increase. The cost of these actions to our society is staggering—not only in the present, but for years to come. Despite our best efforts to develop programs that reduce these behaviors, the involvement of youth in these activities is not abating. Youth are not learning the character-building life skills that will promote good citizenship. Therefore, whether you are a parent, teacher, mentor, coach, or youth program leader, you can use Part II of this guide to teach life skills through the use of various activities that allow youth to practice each of the skills. However, we highly recommend that prior to using Part II to teach youth life skills, you first complete Part I for yourself. This will help orient you to the various life skills, enhance your ability to describe and explain the life skills, and increase your comfort in leading or guiding the activities for developing these life skills with youth. The Guide has one additional very important purpose. We want readers to consider the quality of life they desire. Although quality of life has been defined in numerous ways, we believe that it means the general well-being of a person in terms of happiness and health, rather than wealth. There have been two kinds of well-being discussed in the literature associated with positive human health (i.e., quality of life): subjective well-being (SWB) and psychological well-being (PWB). SWB is comprised of a person's subjectively perceived satisfaction with life. According to Deci and Ryan (2002), SWB is derived from the hedonic tradition of philosophical thought that suggests that happiness or pleasure-seeking is the primary goal of life. PWB, meanwhile, is derived from the eudaimonic tradition of philosophical thought. PWB, according to Ryan and Deci (2001), is considered the result of personal flourishing and the fulfillment of human potential, and is more in agreement with the concept of identity. As identified by Ryff (Ryff & Singer, 2006), PWB was conceptualized as "striving toward excellence based on one's unique potential" (p. 14). Ryff's perspective along with self-determination theory (SDT), developed by Deci and Ryan (2000), and life development intervention (LDI), developed by Danish and his colleagues (Danish, D'Augelli, & Hauer, 1980; Danish & Forneris, 2008; Hodge, Danish, & Martin, 2013), represents the focus of our book.

In 1959, Viktor Frankl wrote what we believe is one of the most important books ever written—Man's Search for Meaning. In it he describes the "will to meaning" as the primary motivation in life--the continual search to find a purpose and meaning for our existence. When asked what he felt was the meaning in his life, Frankl said it was to help others find meaning in their lives. Through this guide, that is our goal. We *want to help you help others to find meaning in their lives by teaching them life skills that will enhance their performance in whatever areas they choose, improve their health, and optimize their quality of life.*

In this guide we define what life skills are and provide the background for a number of life skills. Those presented in this book do not represent the complete universe of life skills, but we have included the life skills we believe are the most relevant for teaching others how to enhance their performance, health, and/or quality of life. It is our hope that you will find the material helpful, can learn the skills, and perhaps even teach others these skills to help develop their capabilities and strengths.

Overview of Life Skills

Life skills are often discussed but rarely defined. We consider life skills to be psychosocial characteristics rather than isolated behaviors, such as learning to manage money or cooking a meal. We have chosen to focus on the term life skills because we are concentrating on the teaching of skills. Life skills are the skills that will enable you to succeed in the world in which you live. They can be behavioral (e.g., communicating effectively with others), emotional (e.g., managing feelings), or cognitive (e.g., making effective decisions), and can be interpersonal (e.g., being assertive) or intrapersonal (e.g., setting goals). Some of the environments (settings or contexts) in which we live and work include families, schools, workplaces, neighborhoods, and communities. Most individuals must succeed (cope with and do well) in more than one environment, and as they become older, their number of environments increases. Individuals in the same environment are likely to be dissimilar from each other as a result of the life skills they have already mastered, their other resources, and their opportunities, real or perceived.

Learning life skills is a behavior-change strategy that differs from other approaches because the focus is on self-directed change. In other words, the focus is not on problems but on developing your capabilities and strengths. It is assumed that you want to, and can take an active role in changing your life. These skills teach you how to "take the reins" in your life and develop personal responsibility for your future. While the idea of taking an active role in one's life can be easily understood, it is not so easily accomplished. Many roadblocks stand in the way. Often new skills must be learned, new information acquired, or new actions taken. But these roadblocks are not insurmountable, although they often seem so at first. Change occurs when you realize that the elimination of roadblocks is under your control. For instance, when you learn how to set goals, you learn that you can approach your life in an active way. This produces a sense of self-confidence and control. As a self-directed person, you can plan ahead to prevent future problems, and as a result, you become an active creator of your own future.

Think of any skill or activity at which you are good—a specific sport, cooking, playing a musical instrument or using a weapon for self-defense. You probably first learned the skills at a basic level. To be good, or even excellent, required patience, practice, and persistence. Learning skills requires that you be active and involved through listening, seeing, and doing. Information describes what to do, but not how to do it. It is simplistic and naïve to assume that we can demonstrate a new behavior because we know what it is; in this guide, we focus on how to do it. We hope you will make that commitment to learn some of the life skills presented in this guide. We will provide the framework and opportunity. The rest depends on you.

Developing Life Skills for Adults
Part One

Identifying Dreams and Setting Goals

Instead of thinking about where you are, think about where you want to be. It takes 20 years of hard work to be an overnight success. — Diana Rankin

Understanding the Relationship between Dreams and Goals

Dreams are what you want for yourself. You can have many different dreams, but the first step in reaching those dreams is to think or reflect on your best possible future—the things you would most like to have happen for you. Dreams represent your best possible self, not what you will settle for. Therefore, when thinking about your dreams it is important not to limit yourself. Although dreams can be abstract and/or seem very distant, they are very valuable because they help provide direction for your life. However, if you want your dreams to come true, it requires more than wishing. You must turn your dreams into goals, as a goal is a dream that you work hard to reach. Activity 1.1 will help you reflect on the different areas of your life and what it would take to reach some of the dreams you have. Remember this program is self-paced so do as much as you can or want to do. Take time to think about the questions and your answers. The process is challenging but should be stimulating. This is not a test; it is an opportunity to learn about yourself and what you want for your life, and then a challenge for you to work toward.

Activity 1.1 Dreams for Goal Setting

Consider the following parts of your life: family, friends, physical and mental health, work, finances, education, and spirituality. Choose three parts of your life that are very important to you and describe your dreams for each of the three 10 to 15 years in the future.

1. _____

_____

_____

2. _____

_____

_____

3. _____

_____

_____

How likely is it that you will reach your dream?

1	2	3	4	5	6	7	8	9	10
Not likely									Very likely

What do you need to do to make your dreams happen?

_____

_____

_____

_____

If you expect to reach your dream, how soon will you reach it?

This year _____? Next year _____? Within 5 years _____?

Within 10 years _____? Whenever I can _____?

Setting Goals

Goals are different from dreams but both are very important. As previously mentioned, dreams should represent your best possible self, whereas goals represent the hard work that is necessary to reach these dreams. To enhance your performance, health, or quality of life, you first must set a goal. Goals provide direction, motivation, and plans for the future. Goals are actions undertaken to reach some desired end, not the end itself. In other words, goals are different than results.

Set a two-month goal related to one of the dreams you have for a part of your life. Why a two-month goal? A duration of less than two months may lead to goals that are not very challenging and will not help you feel as though you are making progress towards becoming your best possible self. A duration much longer than two months may be too long to maintain the energy and commitment needed to achieve the goal. By focusing on something tangible for two months, you will experience a sense of accomplishment and then can set another goal that will get you even closer to your dream.

Activity 1.2 includes 10 questions to help you think about what goal you would like to set for yourself. After completing the 10 questions you can set a two-month goal for yourself.

Activity 1.2 Goal Analysis

Consider these questions as you develop your goal.

1. Of all the different domains or aspects in your life listed in Activity 1.1, what is the one you most want to change?

   _____

   _____

2. How long have you wanted to make this change?

   _____

   _____

3. What have you done, if anything, to make this change?

   _____

   _____

4. Describe a time or situation, if any, in which you came the closest to making this change?

   _____

   _____

5. Describe a time or situation in which you felt furthest from making this change?

   _____

   _____

6. What makes this change important to you?

   _____

   _____

7. Why is it so important to make this change now?

   _____

   _____

8. Is the goal based on (check one):
   a. wishful thinking
   b. overly demanding expectations
   c. irrational needs
   d. realistic interests and expectations

9. What do you gain by making this change?

_____

_____

10. What do you gain by not making this change?

_____

_____

After you have completed the goal analysis in Activity 1.2, write down a two-month goal for yourself.

My two month goal is:

_____

_____

_____

_____

_____

_____

_____

_____

_____

_____

_____

_____

_____

_____

_____

_____

_____

_____

_____

_____

_____

_____

_____

Activity 1.3 Goal Statements

When goals are not positively stated, the focus is on the negative, and considerable energy is wasted trying not to do something. Positive means something you want to do. Stating goals positively helps to create a picture of what you want to do, not what you don't want to do. Goal statements that include words like "not," "avoid," "less than," and "limit" should be changed into positive statements so that you can visualize a goal being achieved. In other words, change "I can't" to "I would like to."

Is your goal positive?

Step 1: Think of your favorite animal. Get a good picture of it in your mind.

Step 2: Now do not think of your favorite animal and count to 10.

Step 3: Were you thinking of your favorite animal when I asked you not to?

Step 4: Now think of winning the lottery and what you would do with the money. Count to 10.

Step 5: Were you still thinking of your favorite animal or winning the lottery? Why? Because you were thinking of something positive.

Which of the following statements is stated positively?

_____a. I do not want to have any more arguments with my spouse or friends.

_____b. I want to earn money so I can go on vacation this summer.

_____c. I want to avoid eating desserts at lunch.

Answer—b

The goal must be *defined specifically and clearly*. Goals that are vague such as "do better" or "improve" do not allow you to know whether the goal has been reached and you have succeeded. Remember a basic rule of psychology, "Success breeds success."

Is your goal specific?

Following are some questions to help you think of the goal in specific terms.

1. What is the action to be taken to reach your goal?
2. When will the action occur?
3. Under what conditions will the action take place?
4. Is there a specific number of times that the action must be taken?
5. When you think of your goal do you use words like "more" and "better?"
6. Is it clear to you when you will have reached your goal?

In each of the following pairs identify the goal that is stated more specifically:

(a) I want to be faster than I was last season.

(b) I will work to improve my time by doing intervals two days a week.

(a) I want to be more organized at work.

(b) At the beginning of each work day I will make a list of the tasks to accomplish.

(a) I want to eat more healthy meals.

(b) I will plan (find a recipe, make a list, and buy the ingredients) for three healthy meals each week.

Answer to each—b

A goal must be *important to you*, at least as important as it is to anyone else. If the goal is more important to others than it is to you, it is unlikely it will be achieved or if it is, it will not feel that important or meaningful. Unimportant goals rarely are achieved. Important goals are want goals; less important goals are should or ought to goals. Therefore, to increase the likelihood that energy will be invested in goal attainment, focus on want goals.

Is your goal important to you?

The following questions will help you think of the goal as important.

1. If the goal was not important to anyone else, would it still be important to me?
2. Is this goal important enough to me that I will work hard to reach it?
3. How will reaching the goal help me (if it helps someone else more than you, it is probably not that important to you)?
4. If I try and succeed, how will I feel?

Imagine the following scenario. You are in a group and each person has to write down a goal that it is important to them. Once everyone has their goal written down, everyone must trade their goal with someone else. Do you think achieving the other person's goal is as important to you as your own goal? Would you be willing to work as hard for that goal as your own?

As previously mentioned, goals are different from results. Goals are actions over which *you have control*. You cannot control other's behaviors, nor can you control the outcome of an activity. You only have control over your own behavior and at best partial control over the results. When your goal statement is really an outcome or result like winning a game or losing weight, it is not really a goal, because you do not have complete control over the outcome.

Is your goal under your control?

The following questions will help you think of the goal as under your control.

1. To achieve the goal, are you the one most responsible for making it happen?
2. Are there factors within the goal that are out of your control (e.g., an outcome or result)?
3. Is your goal more of an outcome/result or a process?

Consider the following example. Many people want to lose weight and make that a goal. However, this is not a goal under their control. Losing weight is an outcome; it is OK to want this outcome but this is a not a goal. The goal has to represent something under your control. Examples of goals include preparing a certain number of healthy meals, going to the gym three times a week, or walking two miles after dinner Monday through Friday.

Making Goals Reachable

You have now set a goal. However, just setting the goal does not automatically mean that you can achieve the goal. A goal that is achievable must be reachable. There are four steps to making goals reachable. Goals must be stated positively, specific, important to you, and under your control.

Activity 1.3 outlines an activity with multiple components. Each component provides a further explanation of the four steps and at the end you will have the opportunity to rewrite your goal, if necessary, to be a reachable goal.

Activity 1.4 Goal Assessment

Is your goal reachable?

Was the goal you set a reachable goal? Did it meet the criteria for a reachable goal (i.e., was it positively stated, specific, important to you, and under your control)? Ask yourself the following and then rewrite your two-month goal to ensure it is reachable.

Is your goal stated positively?

Do you see exactly what you want to be able to do? Have you used words such as "not," "stop," "avoid," or "don't" that make the goal negatively rather than positively stated? If so, restate it so it is positively stated.

Is your goal stated specifically?

Will you know when the goal has been reached? Have you used words like "more," "less," or "better" that do not make the goal specific? If so, restate it so it is specifically stated.

Is your goal important to you?

Is this goal important enough for you to work hard to reach it? Is it a want goal as opposed to a should goal?

Is the goal under your control?

Are you most responsible for reaching the goal? Is your goal more of an outcome/result or a process?

Rewrite your goal so that it is reachable.

_____

_____

_____

_____

_____

Notes

Goal Planning

Always work as hard as you can. Never be satisfied with what you do—strive to make it better. But always recognize your accomplishments. — Unknown

Why Is Goal Planning Important?

Having a goal is one thing; achieving or reaching it is something else. Breaking down a goal into manageable steps helps your progress toward the goal. Planning makes the goal less overwhelming and increases the likelihood of goal achievement. If a goal were so easy to reach that planning was unnecessary, it is likely that it would not enable you to truly become your best possible self.

Goal planning is not complex. It is simply a way to help you break the goal down into more manageable steps. On a scale of 1 to 10 with 1 being "no plan" and 10 being "have a solid plan," how well developed is your plan?

1	2	3	4	5	6	7	8	9	10
No plan									Have a solid plan

Would you like help in developing a plan?

1	2	3	4	5	6	7	8	9	10
No help is needed									Yes, I would like help

If you would like help, continue on with this session; if not, simply review the process of developing a goal ladder in Activity 2.1 and proceed to Session 3.

Activity 2.1 Developing a Goal Ladder

Developing a goal ladder involves five distinct steps. After the five steps are listed there are questions to help you complete the five steps.

Rewrite the goal you set for yourself (making sure the goal has the four components of a reachable goal: positive, specific, important to you, and under your control).

1. List everything you must do in order to accomplish this goal. This step is a lot harder than many realize and may take extra time and thought.
2. Make sure everything you have identified meets the four components of a reachable goal (i.e., positive, specific, important to you, under your control).
3. Put in order all the items identified in the second step and identify a timeline for each item being successfully achieved.
4. Create the goal ladder putting the goal at the top. Make sure the first step or rung on the ladder is easy so you will be off to a good start. Sometimes, it is important to take a break when you are halfway up the ladder to see how much you have accomplished.

Developing a Goal Ladder

1. In the space below write your goal that you have set (remember it should be a goal to reach in two months and it should be positive, specific, important to you, and under your control (revisit Session 1 if necessary).

Goal: _____

_____

_____

_____

2. In the space below, list everything you must do to reach your goal. You should aim to have 10 or more things you need to accomplish to achieve the goal. Also, write down each thing the same way you write a goal: positive, specific, important to you, and under your control. Thinking about the plan counts as something you will need to do and may be your first step.

To reach my goal I must:

_____

_____

_____

_____

_____

_____

3. Make sure these are all positive, specific, important to you, and under your control. If not rewrite them.

_____

_____

_____

_____

_____

4. Then number them in the order in which you expect to achieve them, with #1 being the first step you need to take to achieve your goal, which is also usually the easiest to accomplish.

_____

_____

_____

_____

_____

5. Using the order you just created, fill in the goal ladder below step by step but take note that the first rung is on the bottom (just like a real ladder). For examples, in step 1 (at the bottom) write what you expect to do first, in step 2 write what you expect to do second, and so on. Also, write a target date when you expect to complete each step.

_____

_____

_____

_____

_____

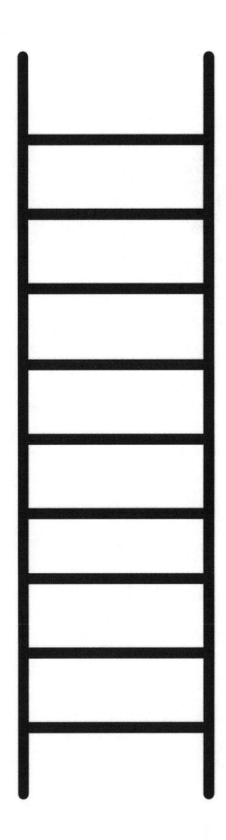

Overcoming Roadblocks to Reaching Goals

Defeat is a lesson for eventual victory. — Unknown

Identifying and Overcoming Roadblocks

A roadblock is anything that may prevent you from reaching a goal. Even when you are committed to achieving your goal it is possible to encounter a roadblock that could prevent you from reaching the goal. There are four main types of roadblocks: lack of knowledge, lack of skill, lack of social support, and fear of failure, which is dealt with in Session 4. The first step in overcoming roadblocks is to identify which of the roadblocks you have encountered.

Lack of Knowledge

You may lack information (facts) that will help you reach your goal. For example, if your goal is to be more physically active, but you are not aware of the types of facilities, programs, or activities that may be best for you, it may be difficult to achieve the goal. To identify lack of knowledge as a potential roadblock, ask yourself the following question: What do I need to know to be able to reach my goal? It may help to review your goal ladder and be sure that you have sufficient knowledge to successfully achieve each rung. If more information is needed, sources such as the Internet, books, brochures, community center resources, online community bulletins, health care providers, family, friends, co-workers, and teachers can help. But remember not all sources are valid and trustworthy. Therefore, check each source for accuracy.

Lack of Skills

You may lack a particular skill or set of skills to reach your goal. Although we most often think of skills as physical, not all skills are physical skills; they may be cognitive skills such as making decisions, or interpersonal skills such as learning to communicate more effectively. So, for example, if you have overcome your knowledge roadblock but now have a choice of two or more programs that will meet your needs for the skills you want to learn, but are also unclear how to perform this physical skill, you have two "how to" (skill) roadblocks—choosing which program (decision-making) and performing the physical skill. Ask yourself the following question: What new ways of acting do I have to acquire to achieve my goal? Once skill roadblocks have been identified, it is important to remember that while knowledge deficiencies may be overcome by identifying resources, most skill deficiencies require practice and feedback. Learning a new skill may require adjustments to the goal and goal ladder. Such adjustments should not be considered a setback but a process that will lead to successful goal attainment.

Lack of Social Support

Another roadblock is lack of social support. You may have the knowledge and skills, but need the support of friends and family to work toward the goal. Just as it is important to have friends in school or in sports who will help and support you, as you work toward your goal you also need that social support. Ask yourself the following question: What reactions, help, and support from others do I need to reach my goal? If this is a roadblock, go to Session 6 and learn about seeking help from others.

Barriers to Goal Achievement

The analysis of roadblocks will help you reflect on barriers you may experience in reaching your goals.

Analysis of Roadblocks Worksheet

1. Do you lack knowledge? Describe what you need to know.

_____

_____

_____

_____

_____

2. Do you lack skills? Describe what you need to learn how to do.

_____

_____

_____

_____

_____

3. Do you lack social support? Describe what support you need?

_____

_____

_____

_____

_____

4. Do you have some combination of a lack of knowledge, lack of skill, and/or lack of social support? Describe.

_____

_____

_____

_____

_____

In addition to reflecting and working to overcome specific barriers, there may also be some additional considerations that are important to be aware of that could prevent you from successfully achieving your goal. First, you may be trying to work on too many goals at once, which may prevent you from having time and energy to focus on any of them. You should work on one goal at a time. Second, if you are not confident in reaching your goal, re-evaluate it and start with one that seems easy and that you are confi-

dent you can achieve. Otherwise, choose to work first on the goal that is most important. Third, if a goal is based on others' expectations, determine if the goal is sufficiently
important to you; if not, forget it. Fourth, if you get stuck working on your goal ladder,
recognize the accomplishments you have made to date and review the step (rung) on
which you are stuck and decide whether the step might be too big or difficult, and if so,
break the step down into two or more smaller, more manageable steps.

Risk Taking to Achieve Goals

What great things would you attempt if you knew you could not fail? — Robert H. Schuller

What Is a Risk?

Risk is an uncertain event that could involve the loss or gain of something you consider to be of value. Formula = Benefits – Costs

Risk Taking in the Goal Achievement Process

The term risk-taking often has negative implications such as behaviors that put our safety at risk (e.g., driving too fast, cliff diving, taking drugs). However, the risk-taking referred to here is not perceived as negative, but potentially necessary to achieve one's goals. You may have all of the necessary knowledge and skills to reach a goal, but be hesitant to take the risk necessary to achieve the goal. Working toward a goal you want is not without emotion. There may be apprehension, hesitation, or fear due to what these changes may bring. There may be worry over whether you can climb the rungs of the goal ladder, fear of failure, or concern about whether taking the risk is worth it. These are all risks.

For example, what if you were considering pursuing a new career? You may know what the new career entails and have the needed skills but are unsure if you will be able to succeed and are afraid to fail because of the possible financial and personal implications. Making a decision to pursue a new career involves change—a big change—since pursuing a new career is not easy. Any time you work toward a goal it means your life changes and the larger the potential change, the greater the risk. With change comes uncertainty, and with uncertainty comes apprehension. Apprehension often leads to confusion about the results of change. There is a tendency to confuse what is likely to happen with what is unlikely to happen.

To determine whether to take a risk, it is important to do an analysis of the risks. An analysis will help you decide, based on your personality and circumstances, whether the goal you have set is worth the risk. When the perceived benefits outweigh the perceived costs, the risks are reduced and the action is worth taking. When the perceived costs outweigh the perceived benefits, the risks are increased and the action is not likely worth taking. The word *perceived* is used because we cannot predict with 100% accuracy the actual costs and benefits. However, even when the perceived costs seem to outweigh the perceived benefits, the goal still may be worth trying to reach. Part of the process of risk-taking is reducing the costs and increasing the benefits, and if this can be done, the goal may be worth keeping, even if it takes a longer time to achieve.

Activity 4.1 Assessing and Taking Risks

Creating a list of pros and cons for a particular goal or rung on your ladder should help you see the benefit-and-cost ratio more clearly. Remember, as you develop your analysis, every action has some advantages (benefits) and some disadvantages (costs). Moreover, for the same behavior, the benefits and costs will likely differ for different people.

For this activity, you will need a dime, a nickel and five pennies or small pieces of candy if these coins are not readily available. You will also need two small envelopes. On one envelope write the word "Completed"; on the other write "Still to do." Once you have all of the materials, work through the following four steps.

Step 1. Assign value to your dreams

From the three parts of your life that were very important to you in Session 1 (Activity 1.1) and for which you described your dreams in the future, assign each a value of 1 to 10 based on how well this part of your life is going right now.

Life Area   Value Between 1 and 10

1: _____   _____

2: _____   _____

3: _____   _____

Step 2. Assign a monetary value to your top three life areas

Choose the most important of the three areas in your life that is not going well and assign it a money value between 1 (penny) and 10 (dime). Describe what would make this area the money value you have assigned, and what has held you back (what risk) from having tried to improve this area. In other words, what actions have you chosen not to do that would make it more valuable, perhaps raising it to a nickel or dime value, if you succeeded in doing it?

Most Important Area:

_____

_____

_____

Step 3: Consider the following questions

What money value are you at now? _____. Put the money you have chosen in the envelope marked Completed.

Now write down what you would have to do to make it a 10, a dime. This is your "to-do list."

_____

_____

_____

_____

_____

What is the best possible consequence if you were to reach a dime and how likely is it to happen?

_____

_____

_____

_____

_____

What is the worst possible consequence if you were to try to reach a dime and failed and how likely is it to happen?

_____

_____

_____

_____

_____

Step 4: Assess the risks
If there are risks involved that prevent you from taking the necessary action, what would you have to do to put the smallest amount in your to-do list? Think of the smallest possible step and even modify your to-do list if necessary.

_____

_____

_____

What action would you have to take, and are there risks in taking just that step? If so, what is the risk(s)? If there are no risks, why have you not already taken this action?

_____

_____

_____

_____

_____

If there is no risk, describe what you will do and by when.

_____

_____

_____

_____

_____

When you complete that step, put a penny in your Completed envelope. Continue to repeat this process while asking yourself the following questions. How much money can you add to your Completed envelope before you identify a potential risk.

_____
_____
_____
_____
_____

What can be gained by taking the next step? How likely is this gain?

_____
_____
_____
_____
_____

What can be lost by taking the next step? How likely is this loss?

_____
_____
_____
_____
_____

If you feel the gain will outweigh the loss, are you ready to take the risk?

_____
_____
_____
_____
_____

If not, is there any way you can reduce the risk and optimize the gain?

_____
_____
_____
_____
_____

If not, then you have gone as far as you can go toward reaching this goal. However, if you have moved closer to the goal as a result of this procedure, you have learned that you can take more risks than you thought and can apply this procedure to other situations and areas of your life.

Notes

Making Effective Decisions

You decide what your life is going to be; you can give up trying or if it is important to you, you can find a way to accomplish it. — Unknown

What Is an Effective Decision?

An effective decision is one that takes in all the possible options, considers them all, and then chooses the one that is the best option. Effective decisions are important because they will help you get closer to your goal and best possible self as well as help prevent roadblocks. Everyday living involves many decisions—a choice to do A or B, or A, B, or C. Some decisions can be minor (e.g., pack a lunch or eat out?), while others are much more serious (e.g., Do I have sufficient training to apply for this new position?). Some people have trouble with minor decisions, but many people experience difficulty in making important decisions, especially when they have to be made quickly with little time to analyze the options. Almost all decisions can be seen in terms of choices: (e.g., Should I reenlist or not? Should I go to graduate school or accept this job offer? Which house should I make an offer for?).

The more difficult the decision, the more overwhelmed one may feel. Some individuals feel overwhelmed and will try to avoid making a decision, or will continually search for additional information to help them with the decision. Regardless, it is important to remember that delaying or choosing not to decide is, in fact, making a decision.

Individuals often make decisions as a result of intuition, reason, or a combination of both. Using intuition is often called using your "gut feelings" and is usually a combination of past experience, emotions, and your personal values. When decisions are being made on gut feelings, it is best to examine these feelings in terms of the emotions, past experiences, and values that are playing a role in the process and determine if they are justified. This is especially important if you have very strong feelings against a particular course of action. See if you can work out why and determine whether your perceptions are accurate. A reasoning approach uses facts and figures to make a decision. However, a reasoning approach tends to ignore emotions, past experiences, or personal values that may affect how a decision is carried out. A more sound approach uses a combination of both intuition and reasoning within a structured approach such as the STAR.

Activity 5.1 Learning About STAR

STAR is a four-step process and stands for Stop, Think, Anticipate, and Respond. This section will help you learn this four-step process and enable you to make effective decisions. You can use the STAR Worksheet at the end of this section to help you work through this activity.

S stands for stop and take a deep breath, or use some other way you have learned to relax yourself. By first relaxing yourself, you decrease anxiety about the decision and can better reflect on any emotions, past experiences, or values that may be involved in the decision-making process.

T stands for think of all your choices or options and all the factors that go into each of those choices or options. For example, if you were considering whether to take Job A or Job B, some of the factors you might consider.

- Job satisfaction
- Relevant past experience
- Financial needs
- Social status needs
- Interest
- Leisure opportunities
- Job security
- Ability
- Need and/or desire for the responsibility of the job
- Needs and/or preferences of family
- Advancement potential
- Geographic preference
- Reputation of the company and alignment of values

A stands for anticipate the consequences of each choice. As part of anticipating, you may want to consider or weigh how each of the factors listed above and any other factors relate to which choice gets you closer to your goals. For example, examine each factor (e.g. job satisfaction) to determine which job choice, A or B, best meets your job satisfaction needs. Continue this evaluation process until each factor is examined. After this process is completed, you should be able to determine which choice will satisfy most factors. For example, an initial weighing of the relevant information might result in:

- Choice A: Factors 1, 3, 4, 5, 6, 8, 11, and 12
- Choice B: Factors 2, 7, 9, and 10

From this weighing process, Choice A satisfies more factors than does B (8 versus 4). Thus, the decision can be made simply on this basis. However, many times the relevant factors are not of equal importance. One factor may be as important, or more important, than all the other factors combined. If this is true, the simple method of evaluation gives too much weight to minor factors. When it happens that one or two of the factors (e.g., factors 9 and 10) are more important than the others, you may want to decide on the basis of which alternative satisfies these important factors.

R stands for respond with the best choice. The best choice is the one that gets you closest to your goal and your best personal self. At this point, you should be able to answer the following two questions:

1. What is my most desirable choice?

_____

_____

_____

2. What is my second choice?

_____

_____

_____

STAR Worksheet

Stop and take a deep breath!

Think—Write down all of the choices.

1. _____
   _____

2. _____
   _____

3. _____
   _____

Anticipate—Write down the factors for each choice. Remember to keep in mind and note accordingly whether the factors have the same importance or whether some are more important than others.

Factors for Choice 1:

_____
_____
_____

Factors for Choice 2:

_____
_____
_____

Factors for of Choice 3:

_____
_____
_____

Are any factors more important than the others?

_____
_____
_____

Respond – Write down the choice you have made.

_____
_____
_____

Notes

Seeking Help from Others: Creating a Social Support Team

Two people are better off than one, for they can help each other succeed. If one person falls, the other can reach out and help. But someone who falls alone is in real trouble. — Ecclesiastes 4: 9-10

The Importance of Creating a Social Support Team

Working towards a goal, changing a behavior, or making a decision can be difficult. Although initiating the process towards a goal or making a change may be exciting, it can be difficult, and maintaining the drive necessary to reach a goal or maintaining change is even more difficult. Most of us can follow our New Year's resolutions—at least for a few days. To change in a lasting way is more difficult. There are no magical ways to maintain new behaviors, but having the support of friends and family often helps. A social support team is a group comprised typically of friends, family, and peers with whom you feel supported and can ask for help when additional assistance is needed. Reaching goals, learning skills, acquiring information, and taking risks all depend to some degree for their success on having a support system, which is a group of others who are important to you and upon whom you can depend. The ultimate source for maintaining a new behavior comes from individuals in your environment. In addition to helping with goal achievement, behavior change, or a life transition, a social support team also provides a number of benefits such as an increased sense of belonging, an increased sense of self-worth, and a feeling of safety and security.

Overview of the Skill

Creating a social support team is different for each person. Some individuals may not need to create a new team because they already have a team that can specifically help them with a particular goal, behavior change, decision, or life transition. Others may have a good social support team but would benefit from adding new members to help them with a particular concern. Finally, some may be experiencing a life event or life transition that has led to the loss of a strong social support team and are in need of strengthening or developing a new team. In addition to creating a new support team, you may need to nurture the relationships with others on your social support team, particularly new members.

The development and maintenance of a successful relationship is a two-way street. The better a friend or support you are to a friend, family member, or colleague the better that friend, family member, and colleague will be to you. Following are some simple strategies that can help remind you how to nurture the relationships you have with members of your social support team.

- Stay in touch. Take the time to return calls and emails as well as offer and accept invitations to do things because this helps people know you care.
- Listen. Find out what is important and going on in their lives and listen to them when they speak to you.
- Celebrate their successes. When someone in your social support team succeeds, celebrate his or her accomplishments.
- Appreciate your support team. From time to time thank the members of your support team for being there for you and express how important they are to you.
- Return the favor. Be there for them when they need support.

You need to be aware that some members of a social support team can be more harmful than helpful. Sometimes a friend may have a different view and may not be helpful in a situation in which support is needed. It is important for you to recognize how a social support team may change depending on the issue. Therefore, a support team may be different for different goals, decisions, or behavior change. Activities 6.1 and 6.2 can help you develop and strengthen a social support team, identify the help needed, and help you communicate that need. Activity 6.1 outlines how one can help further strengthen or create a new support team. Activity 6.2 is intended to help those who have a strong support system but need help identifying how each member of the team may be best able to help, and how to ask for that help.

Activity 6.1 Building Your Social Support Team

There are a number of ways to build a social support team. We recommend a team of about eight individuals. Following are some guidelines to help you decide who may be best to include on the team. Members should be those you see or interact with regularly, who know your strengths and weaknesses, who care about you, and who are willing to help.

You should choose a variety of team members. Some may be family members who provide love, support, and caring; friends or colleagues you trust and spend a lot of time with; and/or individuals who have been important in your life and may serve as role models, such as teachers, coaches, ministers, program leaders, supervisors, and family friends. Once you have begun to identify potential team members you can move on to Activity 6.2, which further helps you identify the type of help each team member can provide and how to seek out that help by communicating with each member of the team.

Activity 6.2 Identifying How Others Can Help

Having a social support team that will function optimally is more than just a process of identifying who is part of the team. For any type of team to function optimally all team members need to know what their role is and what is expected of them. Therefore, you may need to go beyond identifying the individuals who will help and also identify what support or help is needed. There are two kinds of help: caring and doing help. Caring help involves listening and being supportive; doing help involves carrying out a behavior or action. For example, your goal is to return to school there should be members of the social support team that can listen to concerns and provide the emotional support needed in such a transition. There also should be members who can collect information about classes, and/or help you physically move to the school. It is important to recognize that some members of a social support team may only provide caring help, other may only provide doing help, and others may be able to provide both types of help. In the worksheet, you should write down the names of the members of your social support team. Second, identify whether each member can provide caring help, doing help, or both. Third, you should communicate with each team member to explain the help you need and how you think they can contribute. Without such communication it is difficult, if not impossible, for the members to know what is expected of them and how they can be most helpful to you.

Dream Team

List the names of the dream team members. In the second column identify whether they will provide caring support by placing a C, doing support by placing a D, or both types of support by placing a B. In the third column briefly state how they can support you.

_____

_____

_____

_____

_____

Describe what you will say to a potential support team member or members to request that he or she be helpful to you. Write the exact words you will use.

_____

_____

_____

_____

_____

Managing Stress

Much of the stress that people feel doesn't come from having too much to do. It comes from not finishing what they've started. — *David Allen*

Managing Stress

What is stress? Essentially, anything you perceive as a threat to reaching your best self or your well-being. The ability to manage stress is critical because stress can have a number of negative effects on both your mental and physical well-being such as increased anxiety, irritability, forgetfulness, anger, difficulty focusing, burnout, headaches, chest pain, muscle aches, and difficulty sleeping. Also, when stress occurs over a long period of time it can lead to the development of chronic diseases such as heart disease and obesity. Moreover, if you are unaware of how to cope with stress in healthy ways, you may be likely to engage in other behaviors to deal with the stress that further compromise health and well-being such as alcohol or drug use, eating too little or too much, or isolating yourself.

Overview of the Skill

Stress is a normal part of life. Although most people interpret the word stress as negative, stress can also be very helpful. Stress can help you focus and stay alert. Without any stress many believe that our lives are not very engaging. However, as previously mentioned, too much stress can cause difficulties as it can decrease mental and physical well-being. At this point it is important to distinguish the term *stress* from the term stressor. Stress is the feeling of tension we experience, whereas a stressor is the stimulus that causes the stress. While stressors are usually events (e.g., having to plan a family reunion), situations (e.g., going to the doctor), or even another person in your life with whom you have trouble communicating or interacting (e.g., a supervisor, family member), any situation that may lead one to feel stressed can be considered a stressor to that individual. However, it is important to understand that it is not the event or situation inherently that causes stress, it is how you interpret the event. As a result, an event or situation that may be a stressor for one individual could be an event or situation that is enjoyable for another person. In almost any situation, however, if you believe you have the skills or resources to cope with the situation, then it is not likely to cause stress.

To manage stress you need to be able to identify your stressors. To do so it is also important to understand the ABCs of stress. A represents the activating event, B represents the beliefs you feel about the activating event and the resources available to deal with it, and C represents the consequences of the beliefs about the event and your available resources. For example, you have had some tests taken by the doctor and the doctor has called and asked you to come in to talk about the results. The appointment is the activating event. The activating event triggers thoughts, typically based on past or similar experiences, and these thoughts—what you tell yourself about going to the doctor—are the beliefs. What you then feel as a result of your beliefs become the consequences, which may be physiological changes such as sweating and increased heart rate, or emotional changes such as feeling worried or afraid of what the doctor might say. Ultimately, it is also important to remember the fact that everyone will experience stress because it is unrealistic to be prepared or feel prepared to cope with every possible activating event. Another resource that might be helpful in understanding stress and the stress response is a video on the Ted Talk website that describes how the relationship between stress and health outcomes is affected by how you interpret the stress. This talk is titled, "How to make stress your friend," by Dr. Kelly McGonigal.

Activity 7.1 Identifying Your Own Stressors

Following is a Table 7.1 that you can complete to help you identify your stressors. It may be helpful to answer the following questions for each stressor you want to identify, as we all have more than one potential stressor in our lives:

1. Write a brief description of an activating event that led you to feel stress.

_____

_____

_____

_____

2. What did you tell yourself? What were your beliefs?

_____

_____

_____

_____

3. What were the consequences?

_____

_____

_____

_____

4. In the future, how can you change what you told yourself that would lead you to interpret the same situation differently? What can you say or do to help this be a non-stressor?

_____

_____

_____

_____

Table 7.1 Activating Event, Beliefs, and Consequence

A = Activating Event *"Something happens"*	B = Beliefs *"I tell myself something"*	C = Consequence *"I feel something"*
EXAMPLE 1: You are asked to take over a large project at work.	You are not ready for this much responsibility. In your last job you had trouble meeting deadlines when working on larger projects and you are still trying to figure things out at your new job.	Anxious, worry, increased heart rate, and sweaty palms — stress response.
EXAMPLE 2: You and your spouse disagree about how to discipline your child.	You and your spouse have had disagreements on big issues like this one and you have worked them out by communicating openly and finding a compromise or developing a plan that works for everyone.	Assured, confident, empowered — no stress response

The earlier you are able to recognize and understand that how you perceived a situation will determine whether or not a stress response occurs is important. Three points to remember: 1) Different individuals will interpret the same situation in different ways. 2) The ability to interpret a situation as stressful will depend on the resources you have to cope with in that given situation, your past experiences with similar events, and your preparation for the event. 3)Not all individuals have the same resources or skills to cope with different situations.

Strategies for Managing Stress

Another important skill is to develop a way to manage the stress response when it occurs. The management of the stress will decrease the negative symptoms and, in turn, decrease the negative impact that stress will have on your physical and mental well-being. There are a number of ways that you can decrease your stress levels. Four different strategies are outlined that you can learn and use to manage your stress. It is recommended that you practice all four strategies, as different strategies can be used in different situations and also may affect you in different ways. The four strategies are: *breathing*, *progressive muscle relaxation*, *using a mantram*, and *exercise*. Each of the strategies are described and accompany a log sheet that you can use to track progress with the four strategies. Finally, once you have the ability to use all four strategies you will have a greater number of resources to cope with stress and the ability to use the strategy that will be most effective for them in any given situation.

Deep Breathing

1. Deep breathing reduces stress by relieving body tension. Following is a step-by-step process that you can use to master this skill.
2. Begin by sitting erect, but comfortably.
3. Focus on something in front of you or close your eyes and focus on an idea.
4. Place one hand on your abdomen and the other on your chest.
5. Inhale deeply and slowly through your nose into your abdomen (for four seconds). You should feel your abdomen rise with this inhalation and your chest should move only a little.
6. Hold your breath for a couple of seconds.
7. Exhale through your mouth slowly (for four seconds).
8. Practice this breathing activity for two minutes, five times a day for one week. Keep a log of what you have done each day. Use the chart at the end of this Session to log your progress and record how successful you have been.

If you find yourself in a situation in which you do not have a lot of time, take three deep breaths. As you develop the skill you should find that the number of breaths you need to relieve tension will decrease.

Developing a Mantram

A mantram (mantra) is a word or phrase used that helps people relax and find inner peace. Some use a religious or spiritual word, while others use a secular word. When choosing a mantram, it is important that the word or phrase is positive, has no negative associations, is easy to remember, and has a pleasant sound. It is often important that the word has meaning to you.

There are many different ways to use a mantram. The strategy below was shared by Dr. Jill Bormann. That an effective and portable method is silently repeating it during non-stressful, neutral times while disregarding any other thoughts. This practice helps you train your attention and feel calm. Examples of non-stressful times may include waiting in line or before falling asleep. With practice, you can focus on the word chosen and repeat it silently. This will relax you as you mentally repeat the word and disregard any other thoughts, including stressful ones. In other words, it will help reduce stress, increase focus, and transform the way you think. It can be used anywhere, and at any time. Following is a simple two-step process you can use to develop a mantram:

1: Choose a mantram
  - Choose a word or phrase that has meaning and is relaxing.
  - It can relate to a profession, religious or spiritual beliefs, or a word or phrase that has a special peaceful or relaxing meaning such as the name of an important person or thing.
  - Try your word for a few days and see how the word fits. If it does not fit, try another word.
2: Use the mantram
  - Once you have a word that works, start repeating it every day while walking, waiting in line, before going to sleep, while brushing your teeth, or any time to stop ruminating on an upsetting thought.
  - Focus on the word and let any other thoughts disappear. When other thoughts intrude, focus more on the mantram and let the other thought slowly drift away.
  - Over time, you will begin to experience a greater sense of control over your thoughts and feelings, and reduced reactivity to events that generally can cause stress.

Progressive Muscle Relaxation

Progressive muscle relaxation involves tensing and relaxing various muscle groups. When a muscle is tensed and held, the muscle becomes fatigued. When the tension is released the muscle relaxes (becoming even more relaxed than before the tension because the muscle is fatigued). When the body is relaxed, stress is reduced. An important aspect of this exercise is focusing on increasing awareness of the changing levels of tension created by tensing and releasing different muscle groups. When the focus is on the different sensations created by tensing and relaxing the muscles, you will be more aware of rising levels of muscle tension and therefore be better able to monitor levels of tension and do these exercises, before the level of tension becomes excessive. This tension will be a cue to take several deep breaths and relax the muscles that are tense.

When practicing the relaxation exercises try to pair deep breathing and the mantra to enhance the feeling of relaxation or simply think of the word calm. C stands for the chest being relaxed, A stands for arms being relaxed, L stands for legs being relaxed, and M stands for mouth and face being relaxed.

You should work on all of the various muscle groups in the body, one at a time, during this process. Learning this process and doing these exercises is much easier while listening to an audio file. Following is a list of audio files available on the Internet that will make developing this skill much easier. You could also create your own recording or have someone read the script to you.

Textbox 7.1 Progressive Muscle Relaxation

Dartmouth College Student Wellness Center
- https://www.dartmouth.edu/~healthed/relax/downloads.html#muscle

McKinley Health Center – University of Illinois at Urbana-Champaign
- http://www.mckinley.illinois.edu/units/health_ed/relax_relaxation_exercises.htm
- http://www.mckinley.illinois.edu/units/health_ed/stress_audio/PMR%20Head%20to%20toe.mp3

Brigham Young University – Counseling and Psychological Services
- https://caps.byu.edu/audio-files
- https://caps.byu.edu/sites/caps.byu.edu/files/mp3/Progressive%20Muscle%20Relaxation.m4a

Relax for a While Website
- http://www.relaxforawhile.com/visit_joanne_on_youtube/

Inner Health Studio Website
- http://www.innerhealthstudio.com/relaxation-downloads.html

Guided Relaxation – Progressive Muscle Relaxation Video
- https://www.youtube.com/watch?v=2ZKNr-W9A1U

Physical Activity

Physical activity can be described as any activity that uses large muscle groups, that can be maintained continuously, and is rhythmic in nature. Physical activity reduces stress by producing feel-good neurotransmitters in the brain, called endorphins. Additionally, by focusing on the physical activity itself, you forget some of the stresses and your activity improves. Physical activity involves the heart and lungs and causes them to work harder than when at rest. Find something enjoyable that keeps your heart rate elevated for a continuous time period while moving (e.g., walking, cycling, running, swimming, jumping rope, or playing a team sport). However, if you are not currently active make sure to consult with a medical provider or a physical/recreational therapist to see if the workout needs to be adapted. Once you choose the type or types of physical activity in which you wish to participate, make a plan to engage in this physical activity on a regular basis.

Stress Strategies Log							
	Sun	Mon	Tues	Wed	Thurs	Fri	Sat
Breathing (X in box if practiced)							
Success Rating (1-10)							
Comments							
Mantram (X in box if practiced)							
Success Rating (1-10)							
Comments							
Progressive Muscle Relaxation (X in box if practiced)							
Success Rating (1-10)							
Comments							
Physical Activity (X in box if practiced)							
Success Rating (1-10)							
Comments							

Using Positive Self-Talk

When you doubt yourself
It is like joining your enemy's army
And bearing arms against yourself.
You make your failure certain by being
The first person to be convinced of it.
　　— *Adapted from Alexander Dumas*

What Is Self-Talk?

Self-talk represents all of the thoughts that run through our heads, either positive or negative. It can be things we say silently or out loud to ourselves. When self-talk is positive it can facilitate performance and well-being; when it is negative it can impair performance and well-being.

Why Is Positive Self-Talk Important

Whether you are trying to enhance your performance, better your health, or improve your quality of life, how you approach a topic is key. One of the best ways to understand how you respond to any topic is to listen to how you talk to yourself. Everyone talks to themselves all the time. Sometimes we realize it, other times we do not. When self-talk is negative, it hurts us. In contrast to the quote by Alexandre Dumas above, when the self-talk is positive it can facilitate efforts, develop confidence, and lead to greater success.

Overview of the Skill

Everyone engages in self-talk. The key is determining what type of self-talk—positive or negative—you utilize, and under what circumstances you use each type. It is important to recognize that your performance in all aspects of life, as well as your well-being and quality of life, are greatly influenced by your thoughts and expectations, which are usually communicated through self-talk.

Everyone wants to perform well in all the activities in which we participate, including relationships and life. When you set goals, you want and expect to achieve them. When you do not reach them, do you get upset, frustrated and/or angry, berate yourself, lose your temper, and even call yourself names? The anger is directed at you as a person rather than your performance. The result is that the criticism turns into self-defeating thoughts, which make performance worse. Comments such as "I am a lousy athlete," or "I don't know how to talk to people," only reinforce poor performance. Actions mirror thoughts, and the prophecy becomes self-fulfilling. Also, when the focus is inward on you, rather than on your performance, it is not clear how to improve that performance. Therefore, if you do have self-defeating thoughts, you must change that kind of talk to descriptions about how to improve performance. Statements such as "I run like I weigh 800 pounds," or "I play like I have 10 thumbs," should become "I need to relax and concentrate on lengthening my stride," or "I have played this piece many times before. Concentrate on the music, not on who is in the audience."

It is also important to recognize that there are three main types of self-talk: emotional, technical and memory. Emotional self-talk is comprised of statements that generate positive emotions (e.g., the statement "I can do this," often leads to positive emotions such as happiness and confidence) or negative emotions (e.g., the statement, "I am going to fail," often leads to emotions such as frustration, disappointment or anger). Technical self-talk is comprised of statements that either help or hinder you with the execution of a particular skill or behavior ("strong legs, push hard" is a positive example; "don't miss that note" is a negative example). Memory self-talk is a statement made about past events or experiences. For example, when you remember a positive event from the past you may say to yourself, "I have done this before, so I can do it again." If the memory is negative, such as a failed relationship, you might say, "It's not going to work out, just like my last relationship failed."

When thinking about your own self-talk it is important to be aware of the various thinking styles that are considered unhealthy and can lead to increased negative self-talk. Table 8.1 lists some different thinking styles that can lead to negative self-talk.

The following two activities outline a step-by-step approach to help you change your negative self-talk to positive self-talk. It is important for you to understand that changing your self-talk is a skill that involves making and practicing aplan.

Table 8.1 Types of Self-Talk

Types of Self-Talk		
Term	Definition	Example
All or nothing thinking	Sometimes called black and white thinking	If I am not perfect I have failed Either I do it right or not at all
Over-generalizing	Seeing a pattern based upon a single event, or being overly broad in the conclusions we draw	Nothing good ever happens Everything is always rubbish
Mental filter	Only paying attention to certain types of evidence	Noticing only failures and not successes
Disqualifying the positive	Discounting the good things that have happened or that you have done for some reason or another	That doesn't count
Magnification	Blowing something out of proportion, also called catastrophic thinking	If one tiny thing goes wrong, everything will go wrong
Should and must	Using critical words like should, must, or ought; these words can make you feel guilty as if you have already failed	I should practice more I must win
Labeling	Assigning labels to ourselves	I'm a loser I'm completely useless

Activity 8.1 Changing Negative Self-Talk to Positive Self-Talk

Step 1: Recognize Your Self-Talk

The first step in gaining control of self-talk is increasing awareness of what you tell yourself either silently or out load. The best way to recognize and become aware of your self-talk patterns is to keep a log for one week and to write down any negative talk and the context in which it was said. This log should be something you carry everywhere and therefore could be a small notebook or a smart phone.

Step 2: Change Negative Statements to Positive Statements

Once you are aware of your own self-talk, particularly the negative statements, alternative positive ones should be developed. Review your weekly log and write out alternative positive statements that you could have used, noting under what circumstances your self-talk is negative. Once you have gone through all of the statements, pick out a few key statements you believe will work most often. These are the statements to begin practicing. Use the Power Statements box to formulate the positive, affirming statements, called power statements that you can consistently use for your own performance and in your life.

My POWER Statements

1. _____
   _____
   _____

2. _____
   _____
   _____

3. _____
   _____
   _____

4. _____
   _____
   _____

5. _____
   _____
   _____

Step 3: Stop the Negative

Now that you have identified some positive statements, you can begin to practice changing negative self-talk to positive self-talk. To accomplish this change, you need to find a strategy that will help you stop negative thoughts. For some individuals saying something like "stop" or "park it" might work; for others who learn more visually, visualizing a red stop sign may be more effective; and for others who are more active, an action might work best such as placing an elastic (rubber) band around their wrist and flicking the band every time they have a negative thought. You might try all of these strategies and then choose the one that works best for you. Alternatively, create your own personalized strategy to replace the negative statement with one of your power statements. After time and practice, you will likely be able to move away from the general power statements and develop on-the-spot positive statements specifically suited to the situation.

Step 4: Practice Using Positive Self-Talk

Learning a skill, such as changing the way you talk to yourself, is as difficult as learning new physical skills. It involves taking the time to practice it in a variety of situations and being patient. A new skill cannot be learned and immediately applied in every circumstance. As a result it may be helpful to monitor your progress to help recognize the incremental changes you are making. Develop a new log every second or third week and compare these logs to the previous ones. It is important to recognize that all your negative self-talk is not going to disappear in a week, a month, or even a year because it takes time and continual practice. However, the critical point is that you recognize it, work on changing it, and use less negative statements as you proceed through life.

Activity 8.2 Changing Pressure into Challenge

Step 1: Experience a Pressure Situation

Close your eyes and relax by taking several deep breaths. Then visualize a situation in which there are high expectations for you to do well on your performance. Now imagine writing the word PRESSURE across your forehead and assess how your body feels, starting with your arms, face, neck and shoulders, stomach, and legs each for 10 seconds. Gauge your feelings of pressure for each of the different body areas.

Step 2: Relax and Experience a Pleasant Situation

Keep your eyes closed but imagine a pleasant situation such as being on a beach for about 30 seconds.

Step 3: Experience a Challenge Situation

Keep your eyes closed and relax by taking several deep breaths. Then visualize a situation in which there are high expectations for you to do well on your performance, but this time imagine writing the word CHALLENGE across your forehead. Now assess your body, starting with your arms, face, neck and shoulders, stomach, and legs for 10 seconds each. Gauge the feelings of pressure for each of the different body areas.

Step 4: Assessment and Discussion

Open your eyes. Describe whether your muscles felt differently in the pressure as opposed to the challenge situation, and if so, what the differences were and why. If you experienced differences and felt more relaxed in the challenge situation, challenge is a more positive self-talk statement than is pressure. That is because when you feel pressure you are telling yourself you are not sure you can do the performance requested (a negative self-talk statement).

Improving Communication Skills

The single biggest problem in communication is the illusion that it has taken place. — *George Bernard Shaw*

What Is Communication?

The skill of communication enables two or more individuals to converse about topics or issues that have meaning to them, often with the goal of improving relationships. Being able to effectively communicate will be helpful in both developing and sustaining the kind of relationships you want to have with others in your life. For example, effective communication skills can help reduce relationship stress, whether that relationship is with a significant other, friend, or colleague.

Overview of the Skill

Communication is about more than the exchange of information; it involves being able to perceive and understand the emotions being experienced or even the intentions an individual has for sharing particular information. Often times you will say something but others hear something different, and misunderstandings, frustration, and conflicts ensue. Effective communication is how you convey information so that it is received and understood by another person in exactly the way it was intended. It is also how you listen to gain the full meaning of what's being said and to make the other person feel heard and understood. Therefore, improving communication is more than just determining what is said and how it is said. Communication is a two-way street where you have to manage what and how you want to say something as well as how you listen to the other person with whom you are communicating. The easy part is typically figuring out the "what" or content of the message; what is more difficult is the "how" to communicate the message

Like any skill, improving communication requires practice, patience, and a time commitment. To help you improve your communication skills it is important to be able to understand the barriers to effective communication, to learn and practice a variety of communication skills to use on a daily basis, and to also be able to develop a communication plan to address specific topics in a relationship.

You need to understand the barriers to effective communication so that you learn to avoid or overcome these barriers. The first barrier is lack of focus. It is not possible to effectively communicate when you are multi-tasking. If you are thinking too much about what to say, checking text messages, watching a video or show, daydreaming, or thinking of something else, your non-verbal behavior may communicate a lack of attention to the other person. Therefore, the first skill to master is staying focused in the present moment. You can improve your focus by becoming aware of what prevents you from being fully focused. This can be accomplished by understanding the possible distracters (e.g., typing while talking on the phone) when trying to communicate with others. Once you are aware of your common distracters, you can make a plan for how you can stay focused and minimize these distracters.

The second barrier is inconsistent body language. Your nonverbal communication should reinforce or support your verbal communication. You need to be sensitive to whether or how your nonverbal language and verbal language is consistent or inconsistent. To become aware of your nonverbal communication, it is important to have the opportunity to receive feedback in a non-threatening manner or be able to observe yourself. Therefore, having a conversation around the congruence or incongruence observed would be helpful as well as videoing yourself outside the session and having a conversation about what you observed on the videos.

The third barrier is stress or feeling overwhelmed with emotion. When you experience high levels of stress or emotion you are more likely to have a negative interaction with others, such as misinterpreting a situation or message, communicating inconsistent nonverbal language, and/or responding without thinking. You can avoid such situations by recalling past experiences when you have been feeling stressed by doing Activity 9.1 and then using the activities on stress management from Session 7.

Activity 9.1 How Stress Impacts my Communication

In the space provided write down all of the ways that your communication with others is impacted when you're feeling stressed or overwhelmed. What do you do or say that negatively affects your interactions with others.

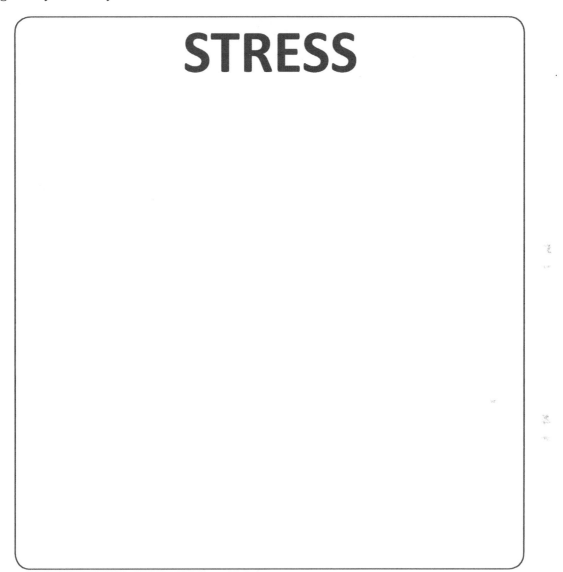

Activity 9.2 I vs. You Statements

As previously mentioned, effective communication is a two-way street. You have to be aware of what you want to say and how you say it, and be open and listen to what another person has to say in return. To reduce the potential for a defensive or angry interaction, you should become familiar with the concept of "I" vs "you" statements. "You" statements (e.g., "You are always trying to argue with me."; "Why do you put down my friends?") shifts blame to the listener, who in return may feel defensive or angry. On the other hand, "I" statements (e.g., "I often feel as if you disagree with my ideas."; "Sometimes it seems to me that you don't like my friends.") allows you to say what you want in an assertive manner, but without making any form of accusation. "I" statements allow you to take responsibility for your feelings and thoughts. Regardless of the situation, "I" statements facilitate positive communication and enhance relationships. It is important to think about when you use "you" statements and practice changing them into "I" statements. Use the worksheet provided to practice this change.

"I" versus "You" Statements Worksheet

In the box provided write out a few statements that you have said to another person in your life that represent a "you" statement or something you would typically say to someone when you are upset about something. Then work on changing each one to an "I" statement. If you have trouble remembering, observe and listen to yourself over the next week and when you find yourself using a "you" statement write it down.

Textbox 9.2 "I" vs "You" Statements

1. "You" or typical Statement:

"I" Statement:

2. "You" or typical Statement:

"I" Statement:

3. "You" or typical Statement:

"I" Statement:

Activity 9.3 Being an Effective Listener

The second part of the two-way street of communicating is to learn to be an effective listener, or what is often called an active or engaged listener. Active listening requires that you not only communicate well, but listen well—not just hear what the other person says but understand the emotions and nonverbal communication of the person speaking. Following are six ways you can increase your listing skills. For those who would like to explore this topic more extensively, refer to Chapters 3 and 4 of our textbook, *Enhancing Performance, Health, and Quality of Life*.

1. **Focus fully on the speaker**, his or her body language, tone of voice, and other nonverbal cues. Tone of voice conveys emotion, so if you're thinking about other things, checking text messages, or doodling, you're almost certain to miss the nonverbal cues and the emotional content behind the words being spoken. Try repeating their words over in your head—it'll reinforce their message and help you stay focused.

2. **Favor your right ear**. The left side of the brain contains the primary processing centers for both speech comprehension and emotions. Since the left side of the brain is connected to the right side of the body, favoring your right ear can help you better detect the emotional nuances of what someone is saying. Try keeping your posture straight and tilting your right ear towards the speaker—this will make it easier to pick up on the higher frequencies of speech that contain the emotional content of what's being said.

3. **Avoid interrupting or trying to redirect the conversation**. For example, saying something like, "If you think that's bad, let me tell you what happened to me." Listening is not the same as waiting for your turn to talk. You can't concentrate on what someone else is saying if you're forming what you're going to say next or trying to redirect the conversation.

4. **Show your interest in what's being said**. Nod occasionally, smile at the person, and make sure your posture is open and inviting. Encourage the speaker to continue with small verbal comments like "yes" or "uh huh."

5. **Try to set aside judgment**. In order to communicate effectively with someone, you do not have to like them or agree with their ideas, values, or opinions. However, you do need to set aside your judgment and withhold blame and criticism in order to fully understand a person.

6. **Provide feedback**. If there seems to be a disconnect between you and the other person, reflect what has been said by paraphrasing (e.g., "What I'm hearing is ..." or "It sounds like you are saying ..." These phrases are great ways to reflect back. Don't simply repeat what the speaker has said verbatim, though—you'll sound insincere or unintelligent. Instead, express what the speaker's words mean to you. Ask questions to clarify certain points (e.g., "What do you mean when you say ..." or "Is this what you mean?")

Activity 9.4 A Strategy for the Tough Conversations

Apart from improving communication on a daily basis, there are times when you need to discuss more serious issues. Following is a step-by-step process to use when having a difficult conversation with an important person.

Step 1: The Planning Phase

Within this phase you should decide on a topic and on a setting for the conversation. It is common and normal for individuals in different relationships to have multiple issues to discuss. Also, it is important to recognize that topics are dependent on the nature of the relationship. Different issues exist when the relationship is between a married couple than it is between a supervisor and supervisee, or an athlete and a coach. For example, for married couples, issues such as money and money management, as well as childrearing may be critical topics, whereas communication style, responsibility, or commitment may be a more significant issue between a coach and an athlete or a supervisor and a supervisee. The time, place, and setting that you choose to communicate is important.

Following are five specific recommendations to help establish a setting that will facilitate an effective conversation.

- Set aside a specific time to talk that works for both parties. Provide an hour for the activity so that neither person feels rushed.
- Avoid having distractions during this time such as supervising children, preparing or tending to a meal, or answering phone calls or texts.
- No alcohol or other drugs should be used before (at least three hours) or during this activity. It is important to remember that this is a time to communicate about important issues.
- Choose a neutral setting that allows both parties to discuss any topic openly and honestly.
- There should be only two people communicating. Third parties may take sides and interfere with the communication.

Step 2: The Interaction

Now that the topic, time, and setting have been established, it is important to interact in a calm and clear manner and be an active listener. Several rules to follow include:

- Make sure to agree on the topic.
- Agree to not interrupt each other.
- Talk in a personal and non-threatening manner, avoiding moral or value judgments. To do this take ownership of what you say by using "I" statements as explained previously.
- Stay on topic. Remember this is the time for both of you to talk. Your job is to respond effectively to what your partner is saying when he or she is talking. Then you should switch and let your partner talk and you listen. Both of you should follow the same rules.

When you are in the listening role there are two rules that should be followed.
- Listen without interruption.
- After the first person finishes talking, the listening person should wait at least 10 seconds and then summarize the content of what has been said. During this process:
- Focus on the important content of the first person's message (not everything said, but the essence of what has been said).
- Summarize the main points in a tentative manner such as saying, "So what you are telling me is" (and then summarize).
- After the summarization, clarify whether the summary was accurate. If it is not accurate, correct any confusion or inaccuracy.
- It may be difficult, but it is important not to be defensive so that the interaction does not become an argument and unproductive.

Throughout the interaction or conversation it is important to be aware of the emotions or feeling being communicated. Recognize that feelings may be expressed verbally or nonverbally. Some individuals can communicate feelings directly, while others cannot. For this reason, listen carefully and be aware not only of what is said but how it is said. If you are unsure about the feeling being expressed, imagine what it would be like to have the feelings about the topic being discussed.

Keep your cool. If you or the other individual become upset or angry, it may be important to take a break. Taking a break may mean going to separate areas of the house, taking a brief walk outside, or having a small snack or something non-alcoholic to drink and deciding when to resume the conversation. Breaks are most appropriate when the two individuals are no longer able to discuss a topic in a calm way and may say or do something either person may later regret. Anger and frustration are normal feelings when trying to resolve differences, so breaks should be limited. However, if possible, before the break begins both individuals should write down where they are (mentally and emotionally). Focus on any feelings, thoughts, or ideas that you have, but are unable to express.

The final aspect to consider is the involvement of other people. Two individuals in a relationship are likely to accomplish more if they are able to keep communication about their problems between them. It is important to acknowledge and recognize that seeking support from others is perfectly acceptable, but substituting the support of a friend or family member to deal with relationships issues rather than communicating directly within the relationship is more likely to hurt rather than help the relationship and the communication process. Allowing more than the two of you to contribute to the communication process may make the conversation one-sided.

Notes

Transferring Life Skills

Ability may get you to the top—it takes character to keep you there. — Unknown

What Does the Transfer of Life Skills Mean?

A skill is not truly a life skill until it is transferred from one domain to another domain. Thus, a skill becomes a life skill when a skill learned in one domain or setting is applied to a new domain or setting. For example, when you learn how to take the skill of setting goals in sport and apply it to school, work, or home, you have learned how to make a skill a life skill.

Why Is Transferring Life Skills Important?

A major roadblock to reaching one's best possible self is either not knowing whether you have the necessary skills or not being able to recognize that some of the skills you have learned in one life domain can be transferred to another life domain. Thinking in new ways about what is already known is part of learning to transfer skills. In fact, it is often not the lack of skills but a lack of knowledge about how to transfer skills from one setting to another that prevents individuals from reaching a desired goal. Understanding what is necessary for skills to be transferable and how one learns to transfer them is an important life skill, and as previously mentioned, is the process of developing your skill set so that you can be more effective.

Overview of Life Skill Transfer

Many researchers with an expertise in life skill development and transfer acknowledge that life skill transfer is not an automatic process. As with any other skill, it takes time and practice. However, the more you work on transferring the life skills you have learned in one life domain to another life domain, the more likely you will experience success in multiple life domains and be closer to reaching your best possible self. Outlined in the following section is a process you can use to help transfer the life skills you have learned to other areas of your life.

The Life Skill Transfer Process

Step 1. You must believe that you have learned a skill or multiple skills that are valued in more than one setting or life domain. For example, if you have too much of your identity tied to one domain (e.g., sport), you may only view yourself as a successful athlete, not a successful person. Such a mindset can rob you of the confidence to try something new or recognize how the skills developed as an athlete may also apply outside of sport. If you do not think you can be successful in other settings, it is unlikely that success in a different setting will occur. Therefore, it is important to become aware of how various skills you have learned in one domain may transfer to another domain. To do this, think about a skill you have recently learned, even one from this book, and write down how this skill may be useful or valued in other domains in your life (e.g., school, work, sport, home, friends, and community).

Step 2. Once you are able to recognize that the skills you have learned will be quite valuable and useful in multiple life domains, it is important to assess how confident you feel about transferring the skill. If you do not feel confident about the transfer process, you need to recognize other times that you have successfully transferred some type of skill from one domain to another. Using an easy example will help you recognize that in the past you have been successful in transferring skills from one domain to another and that you can transfer life skills with little guidance and support. Identify one skill you learned in a domain such as school or work, and where else you have applied this skill.

Step 3. Now that you have recognized one skill that you have successfully transferred, think of two or three more. Again, the skills transferred do not have to be complex (e.g., learning how to work with your peers at school allowed you to be able to work on a project with a new colleague; learning how to manage your time between classes, training, and work at your university allowed you to manage your time between work, family, and your community commitments). Overall, the purpose of this is to help you recognize that we all have skills, both simple and more complex, that we have learned or can learn to transfer to other domains.

Step 4. Once you have successfully identified how you have transferred some of the skills you have learned in the past to a different domain, you can use the Life Skills Transfer Worksheet to reflect on how you can transfer each of the life skills that were covered in this book or other life skills you have learned in other domains that you believe would be valuable in different domains. You may also find it helpful to use the section that is presented after the worksheet; it outlines concrete examples of transfer for all of the skills in this book. Remember, by engaging in life skills transfer you are not only strengthening the development of that particular skill but also getting closer to your personal best in all the various domains in your life.

Life Skill Transfer Worksheet

What Life Skill do I want to transfer?

_____

_____

_____

_____

To what life domain do I want to transfer the skill?

_____

_____

_____

_____

How has this skill helped me so far?

_____

_____

_____

_____

How will transferring this skill help me?

_____

_____

_____

_____

What steps do I need to take to transfer the skill?

_____

_____

_____

_____

Transfer of Goal Setting

To become your best possible self it is likely that you will need to set goals in multiple areas of your life. Following are concrete examples as well as some questions to help you facilitate the transfer of goal setting into multiple life domains. Concrete examples: Work–Set a goal to accomplish a particular project. School–Set a goal to understand a particular concept with which you are having difficulty. Home–Set a goal to help everyone be more physically active. Social Life–Set a goal to spend more quality time with friends and family. Performance–Set a goal to master a particular skill or technique.

Questions that can facilitate transfer:
- Do you have ideas of what your best possible self may be in other areas of your life (e.g., work, school, family, friends, community)
- Do you think the skill of goal setting could help you become your best possible self in these other areas?
- What dreams or visions of your best possible self do you have for different areas of your life?
- Are there any goals you could set now to help work towards one of those other dreams?

Transfer of Goal Planning

The skill of goal planning that you learned as part of creating a goal ladder is transferable to many areas of life and can help you succeed in achieving a number of outcomes. Following are a number of concrete examples as well as questions to facilitate the transfer of goal planning in other areas of your life. Concrete examples: Work–Create a goal ladder for your goal to finish a major project that you have been asked to undertake by your supervisor. School–Create a goal ladder for your goal to feel prepared for your final exam. Home–Create a goal ladder to complete a project at home that has been on your "to do" list. Social Life–Create a goal ladder to help you reach your goal of being more involved in the community. Military–Create a goal ladder to increase your strength and agility.

Questions that can facilitate transfer:
- What major projects that you know will take some time have been on your "to-do" list for a while? (e.g., work, school, family, friends, community)?
- Do you think the skill of goal planning can help you achieve some of these major projects?
- What project on your "to-do" list do you think would be best to use a goal ladder to accomplish?

Transfer of Overcoming Roadblocks

You will likely face roadblocks in all areas of your life at some point or another, so being able to transfer this skill to multiple domains is valuable. Following are a number of concrete examples as well as questions to work through to help facilitate the transfer process. Concrete examples: Work–Developing a particular skill that you need to achieve so that you can be promoted. School–Asking a professor for help to understand a new concept. Home–Asking a significant other to help more to better manage the household responsibilities. Social Life–Gaining more information on community events and activities to broaden your social network. Performance–Developing a particular skill that will help your reach a goal.

Questions that can facilitate transfer:
- Are there potential roadblocks that currently exist in your life that are preventing you from being your best possible self?
- What are these roadblocks that may be contributing to a lack of progress on projects that have been on your "to-do" list for a while? (e.g., work, home, school, community)
- What other roadblocks do you think you could overcome with these strategies?

Transfer of Risk-Taking to Achieve Goals

It is important to recognize that risk-taking can be helpful in multiple domains to either achieve a goal or make a decision. Following are some concrete examples and questions you can use to help begin the process of transferring this life skill. Concrete examples: Work–Weighing the potential benefits versus the costs of confronting a supervisor about unfair treatment in the workplace. School–Thinking about the pros and the cons about taking what are known as "easy" courses versus courses that might challenge you more. Home–Determining the benefits and costs of implementing new household rules to equalize responsibilities. Social Life–Whether to end a relationship that you are not finding to be a positive influence in your life. Performance – Whether to keep training and competing or retire.

Questions that can facilitate transfer:
- Are there other life domains in which taking a risk to reach your best possible self may be worth considering?
- What life domain would this be?
- Do you think using a pros and cons list could help you determine whether to take a risk in another life domain?

Transfer of Making Effective Decisions

Effective decision making is a life skill that can also be used on a daily basis in every domain of life. Therefore, it is important to recognize how to use the STAR approach for any decision you make. Following are a number of concrete examples and questions to facilitate the process of transfer of effective decision making. Concrete examples: Work–Whether to apply for a new position. School–What courses you will need to be able to obtain a particular certification or entry into a post-graduate program. Home–

Whether to sell your house and look for a new one or renovate the one you have. Social Life–Whether to move to a new city. Military–Whether to re-up.

Questions that can facilitate transfer:
- Are there decisions that have been weighing on your mind that you should make?
- Do you think using the STAR approach could help you make some of these decisions?
- What decision would you like to tackle first?
- How could you help others in your family or social network use the STAR approach in their lives?

Transfer of Seeking Help from Others

Developing a strong social support team is important for positive functioning in all life domains. You need to develop a strong social support system to succeed in reaching all your goals in multiple life domains. Following are a number of concrete examples as well as questions to work through to help facilitate the development of multiple social support teams. Concrete examples: Work–Identifying a core group of colleagues that can support you in completing a major project. School–Having a peer or group of peers that can help you achieve your academic goals. Home–Establishing a group of family members and/or neighbors that you can rely on for support for aspects related to a family member's illness. Social Life–Developing a small group of close friends that you can rely on for doing an activity you enjoy (e.g., a sport team, a book club, a dinner club). Performance–Developing a core support crew that may consist of your coach(es), teammates, health professionals, or family that can all provide support to reach your performance goals.

Questions that can facilitate transfer:
- Are there other life domains in which enhancing your social support team would help develop your well-being?
- What life domain or domains would this be?
- Do you think identifying potential members of this social support team or teams would be a good first step?

Transfer of Managing Stress

Similar to developing a strong social support team, coping effectively with stress by developing stress management strategies for one particular life domain or for strategies that may work effectively in multiple domains is important. Following are a number of concrete examples as well as questions to work through to help facilitate the transfer of stress management techniques to multiple life domains. Concrete examples: Work–Going to work or being at work causes increased tension due to various factors such as tight deadlines, overbearing supervisor, or tensions with colleagues. School – Increased stress and tension when writing an exam. Home–Feeling overwhelmed trying to keep up with responsibilities at home and outside the home. Social Life–Ongoing conflict among friends or family members. Performance or Military–Increased stress when competing, particularly at important events.

Questions that can facilitate transfer:
- Are there other life domains in which the stress management strategies you have been practicing will help decrease stress?
- What life domain or life domains would this be?
- What stress management technique would work best in this situation?

Transfer of Positive Self-Talk

Positive self-talk is a skill that you should be using all of the time in all domains of life. It is important to learn how to change negative self-talk to positive self-talk. Sometimes negative self-talk is used in general, and sometimes it is specific to a situation. Either way, it is important for you to increase your positive self-talk. As with the skills discussed previously, following are some concrete examples and questions to help facilitate transfer of positive self-talk. Concrete examples: Work–Talking negatively to yourself about whether you will get an upcoming promotion. School–Engaging in negative self-talk when doing math homework. Home–Thinking you are not a "good enough" parent, provider, or significant other. Social Life–Doubting why friends want to spend time with you or doubting your contributions to existing friendships. Performance or Military–Talking negative to yourself about your performance at a recent event/competition or testing event.

Questions that can facilitate transfer:
- When do you use negative self-talk? Does it occur more often in some life domains than others?
- If so, what domain does it occur in most?
- How can you change your negative talk into positive talk in all domains of your life?

Transfer of Communication Skills

Communication, like positive self-talk, is a skill that you can use in all domains of life. Being an effective communicator is helpful in one-to-one interactions as well as in general with all people. As with the skills discussed previously, following are some concrete examples and questions to help facilitate transfer of communication skills. Concrete examples: Work–Improving communication with a colleague in which there is tension. School–Improving communication with your friends. Home–Improving communication with your significant other or children. Social Life–Improving communication with a friend or an extended family member. Military–Improving communication with your unit.

Questions that can facilitate transfer:

- Is there another person in your life with whom you wish you had better communication? How would you like to see that communication improve?
- Would the use of more "I" statements help in this situation?
- Can the step-by-step process you learned previously help you in your communication with this person?

Preparing for Life Transitions

The future belongs to those who believe in the beauty of their dreams. — Eleanor Roosevelt

What Is a Life Transition?

A life transition is any period of time when you experience a significant change in your day-to-day living. Such transitions are usually preceded by a critical life event. Some of these life transitions are those expected to occur and can, to a certain extent, be planned for; others can occur unexpectedly; and occasionally a life transition we expect to occur does not happen. The concept of critical life events is especially important during the second half of life, as a part of adult development (e.g., changing family situation or employment, changing economic resources). However, these changes are more than discrete events. They should be considered as processes, beginning well before the event occurs and continuing beyond when the actual event has happened (e.g., getting married). This life skill will be especially relevant if you are planning or have recently begun a life transition or if you have experienced a sudden unexpected life event that has led to changes in your life situation.

Preparing for Life Transitions an Important Part of Developing Life Skills

We experience many transitions during our lifetime. In order to successfully navigate these multiple transitions, it is important to be aware of possible upcoming transitions as well as to be as prepared as possible for their occurrence. Prior to starting preparations it is imperative to recognize five factors that play a role in whether a life transition is more easily negotiated or may pose more of a challenge. These five factors include the following:

Timing relates to social or personal expectations of when an event occurs relative to when the life transition is expected. For example, retirement at 35 is "off time" but at 65 is "on time." When an event or transition occurs "on time" you are usually better prepared and have less difficulty successfully navigating through the transition.

Duration relates to the length of time the event or transition is experienced. In general, the longer a transition takes the more resources are required; therefore, the ability to cope with the transition may be more difficult. On the other hand, if a transition occurs very suddenly and is short in duration, you may have difficulty, given that you may not have had sufficient time to effectively cope with rapid changes during such a transition.

Sequence relates to whether the event or transition occurs in the expected societal or personal order. For example, it is common to see the following pattern—a relationship with a significant other begins, a career starts, marriage/commitment to a significant other follows, children are born and raised, career advancement occurs, followed by retirement. When a life transition occurs out of sequence, you may experience difficulties coping as a result of lack of social support or lack of reliability of others and/or other resources that are typically in place to help you work through the traditional sequence of life events.

Contextual purity relates to the extent to which a life event or transition interferes with the resolution of other events. When more than one event occurs at the same time, such as having a child and an opportunity for career advancement, the coping process may be more difficult as you are dealing with two transitions relatively simultaneously.

Probability of event occurrence relates to the probability (either high or low) of an event occurring for a large percentage of the population. When you experience a life transition that often occurs to others, you are also more likely to be able to successfully navigate through this life change. This is because you have observed others navigating the same or similar transition.

Overall, when a life transition is off time, has a long duration, is out of sequence, interferes with other events, and/or is unlikely in regards to probability there is a greater chance that you will experience the transition as a disruption in your life rather than an opportunity for personal growth. However, by being aware of these noted factors and being prepared, you can turn the transition into an opportunity for personal growth.

Following is a two-step process that you can use to help enhance the chances of the various life transitions being experienced as opportunities for personal growth.

Step 1. Exploring the factors related to the transition

The first step is to assess how the five factors are going to affect you. Consider each factor and how you feel about the change or process of change resulting from the life transition and identify the resources available to help you successfully navigate the transition.

Step 2. Understanding values and relevant past experience related to the transition

The second step involves examining the life transition in more detail. More specifically, you should reflect on your strengths, personal values in relation to the life transition, and similar experiences that may help you navigate through the transition. The following three activities are designed to help you in preparing for life transitions. We have chosen to make the activities specific to beginning or changing a career (e.g., graduating from college and seeking employment or wanting to make a career change), as this is a very common life transition. However, you could easily adapt these activities by changing the wording in the activities to be more relevant to the life transition for which you want to plan and prepare.

Activity 11.1 What Am I Good at and Enjoy?

Complete Table 11.1 by writing out what it is you enjoy and don't enjoy and what you perceive you are good and not good at.

Table 11.1 Enjoyment Assessment

Things I am good at and enjoy	Things I enjoy, but am not good at
Things I am good at, but don't enjoy	Things I do not enjoy and am not good at

Activity 11.2 My Work Values

The second activity is a values assessment related to the life transition. Read through the various aspects or components of a job and rate each of them in terms of importance. Then prioritize your values and identify positive and negative attributes of previous experiences.

Work Values Assessment

Part A: Identifying Values. Read through each item in Table 11.2 and place an X in the box that best represents how important that item is to you in a work environment.

Work Value	Very Important	Moderately Important	Somewhat Important	Not Important
Being productive				
Making money				
Being able to improve				
Working by myself				
Experiencing success				
Creating something				
Regular travel				
Flexible work hours				
Being my own boss				
Opportunity to supervise others				
Having a chance for personal development				
Helping others to work together				
Owning and running my own business				
Gaining a sense of responsibility				
Working on projects as a member of a team				
Being supervised by someone I respect				
Good benefits package				
Having a variety of activities				
Making new friends				
Working independently				
Being able to make a difference for others				

Table 11.2 My Work Values (continued)

Achieving visibility and fame				
Developing an identity				
Doing something enjoyable				
Challenging myself				
A regular routine				
Working close to home				
Never having to work on weekends				
Never having to bring work home				
Learning my limits				
Job security				
Working with my hands				
Work involving writing				
Work I can do past age 65				
Convincing others to do/buy something				
Opportunity for advancement				
Opportunity to advance in an organization				
Good vacations				
Supportive coworkers				
Pressured work environment				
Opportunity for professional activities				
Company pays for education				
Being loyal to an organization/company				
Working primarily outdoors				
Working primarily indoors				
Work where I can use physical skills				
Work where I primarily use mental skills				
Being able to work on a project over time				
Work that I can complete by the end of the day				

Part B: Prioritizing the Values. From the list of very important work values, choose the 10 most important values for you.

1. _____
   _____

2. _____
   _____

3. _____
   _____

4. _____
   _____

5. _____
   _____

6. _____
   _____

7. _____
   _____

8. _____
   _____

9. _____
   _____

10. _____
    _____

Part C: Assessment of Past Experience. Think about what you enjoyed and disliked about previous volunteer activities, internships, or jobs you have had. In Table 11.3, list the positive and negative aspects.

_____
_____
_____
_____
_____

Table 11.3 Positive and Negative Aspects

Positive Aspects	Negative Aspects

Put an asterisk (*) by any positive aspects you would need to have as part of a new career or job. Put an X by any negative aspects that you would not want to be part of any new career or job.

Activity 11.3 The Million Dollar Question

This activity is intended to help you reflect on what is important to you. It involves asking yourself the "million-dollar question." Doing so will help you identify gaps between your current situation and your ideal situation as well as recognize the potential roadblocks to achieving your ideal situation and how these roadblocks may be surmounted.

Consider the following example. Someone offers you $10 million dollars ($10,000,000). The only thing you have to do for the money is to work at least 30 hours a week. It can be at any career, job, or activity (such as going back to school) that you want and since you do not need to get paid, you are assured of being able to do whatever it is. What will you be doing?

_____

_____

_____

_____

Next, describe in detail what you would want to do with that 30 hours.

_____

_____

_____

Now ask yourself the following questions and if you find it helpful, write down the responses to these questions.

1. How is it different than what you are doing now?

   _____

   _____

   _____

2. What is, or will be in the future, preventing you from having this career or job? What are the roadblocks?

   _____

   _____

   _____

3. How can you overcome the roadblocks? If you need to, revisit Session 3 of this book about overcoming roadblocks.

   _____

   _____

   _____

Notes

Life Skill Evaluation

Session 12 Life Skill Evaluation

We want you to see what you have learned, so we have developed two questionnaire-type evaluations. The first evaluation is specific to the life skills we have taught and will help you assess the areas you feel you have developed and potentially some in which we may want to focus on for further development.

Evaluation 1: Life Skills Assessment

Please read each of the following items and on a scale of 1 to 7, where 1 is strongly disagree and 7 is strongly agree choose the response that best represents you. It is important to be honest with yourself, as being honest will help you to truly evaluate progress over time. If you are able to answer either 6 or 7 on each item, congratulations. If you score under 6 on some of the questions this is completely normal and acceptable, as it takes time to develop skills. The next step is to decide which of these you want to improve upon; you can return to the activities and keep practicing. Remember, becoming your best possible self is a life-long endeavor and the more you develop a variety of life skills the more you will achieve.

1. I know how to set achievable goals.

1	2	3	4	5	6	7
Strongly disagree			Neither agree or disagree			Strongly agree

2. I know how to develop a goal ladder to help me reach my achievable goal.

1	2	3	4	5	6	7
Strongly disagree			Neither agree or disagree			Strongly agree

3. I know how to identify and overcome any roadblocks preventing me from reaching my achievable goal.

1	2	3	4	5	6	7
Strongly disagree			Neither agree or disagree			Strongly agree

4. I know how to assess and take the necessary risks to succeed in reaching my achievable goal.

1	2	3	4	5	6	7
Strongly disagree			Neither agree or disagree			Strongly agree

5. I know how to make effective decisions.

1	2	3	4	5	6	7
Strongly disagree			Neither agree or disagree			Strongly agree

6. I know how to create an effective social support team.

1	2	3	4	5	6	7
Strongly disagree			Neither agree or disagree			Strongly agree

7. I know how to support and take care of others as well as the greater environment in which we live.

1	2	3	4	5	6	7
Strongly disagree			Neither agree or disagree			Strongly agree

8. I know how to manage my stress effectively.

1	2	3	4	5	6	7
Strongly disagree			Neither agree or disagree			Strongly agree

9. I know how to use positive self-talk.

1	2	3	4	5	6	7
Strongly disagree			Neither agree or disagree			Strongly agree

10. I know how to improve my communication skills.

1	2	3	4	5	6	7
Strongly disagree			Neither agree or disagree			Strongly agree

11. I know how to enhance my performance, health, and quality of life.

1	2	3	4	5	6	7
Strongly disagree			Neither agree or disagree			Strongly agree

Evaluation 2: Components of a Successful Person

Being able to succeed in life requires not only understanding a number of life skills and applying them to your life situation, but also having the confidence that you can use them in a number of different situations. Remember, life skill development is an ongoing process and there are always areas upon which to improve. Following are questions that fall within the various areas of becoming a successful person. Read through each question, reflect on the question, and then identify areas of strength and areas in which you need to improve. Once you have identified areas to work on you can continue to practice the life skills you feel will help you improve or enhance this area of your life.

Overall Self Evaluation

- What areas of your life have you identified (or received feedback from supervisors, colleagues, coaches, or teachers) as areas of strength?
- What areas of your life have you identified (or received feedback from supervisors, colleagues, coaches, or teachers) as areas for improvement?

Mental

- Do you have life goals?
- How focused are you?
- Do you have a plan to reach your goals?
- How confident are you that you can achieve your goals?
- Are you able to be "in the present" when you need to be?
- Are you able to separate your self-talk so that the self-talk is on your behavior or performance and not about you as a person?

Emotional

- Are you able to have fun when you practice, work, and/or participate in activities?
- Are you able to choose your attitude?
- Are you able to balance the various aspects of your life—your performance areas, family, friends, school, work, spiritual, relationships, and social life?
- Do you know how to relax?
- Are you able to manage your emotions—be excited, hurt, calm, disappointed, upset, ready, etc.—and show it when each emotion is appropriate?

Social

- Are you able to offer support to others, even to the point of "making someone else's day?"
- Are you able to seek support from others?
- Are you able to communicate effectively?
- Are you able to give and receive feedback?
- Do you work well with others?
- Can you appreciate others even if they are different from you?

Physical
- Do you consume a healthy, varied diet?
- Do you get at least seven hours of sleep per night?
- Do you engage in regular physical activity year around?
- Are you able to maintain a healthy weight?

Conclusion

You have now reached the end of our self-guided activities. We hope you have discovered new ways of thinking and the tools that will help you reach your goals and become your best possible self. We encourage you to return to these activities as needed as practicing these skills will further enhance your confidence and abilities. In addition, as mentioned above, this our attempt at "giving psychology away" and because we believe in social action, we hope that you will share your newly-gained knowledge and skills with others you care about—family members, friends, individuals with whom you care about. Most of us seek out friends, family and neighbors when we are bothered by everyday problems rather than seek professionals. By being a good listener and someone who is knowledgeable about life skills, you become a valuable community resource.

Notes

Teaching Life Skills to Youth
Part Two

Character-Building Life Skills for Children and Adolescents

So far our efforts have focused on enhancing performance, health and quality of life for adults, but we are equally concerned about children and adolescents—how to promote their development as well. Although we will use the term *youth*, our focus will be on ages 6 to 18. In this section, we will: 1) define youth development; 2) talk about people and settings in which youth development can be promoted, namely, at home with parents, at schools with teachers, at religious institutions with clergy, and in extra-curricular activities with coaches and older peers; 3) the barriers that exist within each setting and for each of these groups of individuals; 4) describe a program to promote youth development; and 5) provide training for the individuals in these different settings on how to implement such programs.

Youth generally take more risks with their health, their lives, and their future. Involvement in health-compromising behaviors such as drug use, unprotected and unsafe sex, violent and delinquent acts, and dropping out of school, are a few examples of risky behavior youth may ingage in. The cost of these actions to our society is staggering, not only in the present, but for years to come. Despite efforts to develop programs that reduce these behaviors, the involvement in these activities is not abating. As William Raspberry, a deceased Pulitzer Prize winning columnist wrote: "Too many young people—including some with the potential to elevate themselves, rescue their families, or change the world—allow themselves to be dragged down by the curse of low expectations." Often young people lack the opportunity to be taught how to succeed and as a result give up on school and their future. They fail to learn the character-building life skills that will promote good citizenship. Although many youth development experts look to prevention programs as the answer, we believe that a major focus of working with youth should be to develop competence and promote positive development.

Defining Youth Development

For some, youth development refers to the elimination of problems. However, defining everything in terms of problem reduction is limiting. We do not assess people in terms of problems, or lack of problems, but in terms of their potential. Being problem-free is not the same as being competent or successful. Therefore, we must define and teach youth the skills, values, attitudes, and knowledge necessary to succeed. Numerous organizations have identified competencies related to positive youth development. For example, in a series of reports the Carnegie Council on Adolescent Development identified a number of desired youth development outcomes. In 1989, the Council identified five desired outcomes: (a) the ability to process information from multiple sources and communicate clearly; (b) to be enroute to a lifetime of meaningful work by learning how to learn and therefore being able to adapt to different educational and working environments; (c) to be a good citizen by participating in community activities and feeling concern for, and connection to, the well-being of others; (d) to be a caring and ethical individual by acting on one's convictions about right and wrong; and (e) to be a healthy person. In 1995, the Council identified others associated with personal and social development. They include: (a) finding a valued place in a constructive group; (b) learning how to form close and lasting relationships; (c) feeling a sense of worth; (d) achieving a reliable basis for informed decision-making, especially on matters of large consequence; (e) being able to use available support systems; (f) having a positive future orientation; and (g) learning respect (Carnegie Council, 1989; 1995).

Other researchers and groups identified other desirable outcomes. Pittman (1996) focused on the motivation to be competent in academic, vocational, physical, emotional, civic, social, and cultural areas. Bloom (2000) delineated the needed competencies as the ability to work well, play well, love well, think well, and serve well. We added "be well." Earlier we defined competence as the ability to do life planning, be self-reliant, and be able to seek help from others. With such competencies youth will be better be able to develop confidence in the future, acquire a sense of personal control over themselves and their environment, and to become better citizens. It is our belief that it is the development of life skills that allows youth to thrive and develop these identified competencies that will enable them to succeed in their lives.

Part II of this guide outlines a step-by-step approach for teaching a variety of life skills to youth. In addition, the life skills are broken down into sessions so that you can customize a program for the group or individual youth with whom you are working. Depending on the type of youth life skills program being implemented, the length of the program will vary, but the teaching of the life skills alone will require approximately 30–40 minutes for each skill.

Teaching life skills to youth can be incorporated into an existing program, and in our experience goes hand-in-hand with various sport and physical activities (e.g., basketball, soccer, volleyball, dance, martial arts, golf, cooperative games). When integrated or combined with a sport or physical activity program, a series of stations are often developed to manage larger groups. At one station the participants practice the sport skill or physical activity, at another station the life skills are taught, and at a third station youth participate in the sport or physical activity and the life skills are reinforced. If you have a smaller group, you may want to teach the life skill to everyone at the start of the session and then use a sport or physical activity component for the remainder of your session to reinforce the life skill being taught. However, it should be noted that the life skills can also be taught in a non-sport and physical activity program in which the focus is only on youth learning the life skills. The following section outlines how to teach life skills, how to manage a group, tips on how to provide feedback and implement effective life skills sessions and provides an overview of the different life skill sessions.

How to Teach Skills

Teaching a skill is different from teaching facts and information. Imagine teaching someone how to drive a car or play a sport by having them read a book. I'm sure you wouldn't want to ride in a car with someone who had read a book about driving but had never driven. Successfully teaching a skill requires knowing the skill, understanding the importance of the skill, and demonstrating the skill.

Naming and Describing the Skill

This allows another person to begin to develop a mental picture of the skill. For example, picture what it would be like if you were an athlete and your coach told you to run a new play that you had never heard of before; you would have no idea what was expected of you. But if the coach described the play and gave it a name, you would begin to form a mental picture of the play. The same is true here. You must help youth develop a mental picture of the skills you are going to teach by labeling and describing the skills.

Understanding the Reasons for Learning the Skill

Again, think of learning a new play. You would feel more motivated to learn the play if the coach told you it took advantage of a weakness of your opponent. You would then see why the play was necessary. You might even try to work extra hard on the play because you could see how useful it might be. If youth can see how learning skills will help them, they will be more motivated to learn the skills.

Demonstrating and Practicing the Skill

A skill must be *seen* and *heard*. When you demonstrate a skill you have already named and described, the participants see and hear the skill and form a mental picture of the skill. The skill must then be practiced.

Let's go back to the example of the play again. If the coach demonstrates the play by having another player run it while you watch, you get a clearer picture of what the play involves. You can then try to run the play. However, you're not likely to run the play well the first time. You will be able to run the play well only after you practice the play over and over again. The youth you teach will need to see and hear the new skills that you present. Examples that you give about your experiences *demonstrate* the skill. Then they must *practice* these skills. In fact, the most important part of teaching skills is having an opportunity to practice the skills correctly.

The discussions and activities that take place during the session will provide opportunities to practice the new skills. You should also encourage the youth to practice these skills in their everyday lives, as this will help them transfer the skill, which ultimately takes a skill from being just a skill to a *life skill*.

How to Encourage Discussion with Youth

Three important skills you must learn are: using open-ended questions, rephrasing and reflecting upon the comments made by youth, and including personal examples.

Open-ended questions, unlike closed-ended questions, encourage discussion. They encourage a person to say more about what he or she is thinking or feeling. Open-ended questions cannot be answered with a simple yes or no. They usually begin with the words how and what. Examples of open-ended questions are: "William, how have you been able to set a goal?"

Closed-ended questions don't encourage discussion. Usually these questions begin with words like *did, where, when, are, will,* etc. and can usually be answered with a yes or no.For example, the question, "Juan, did you decide on a goal that you want to work on?" can be answered with a simple "yes" or "no." Because the participant doesn't have to say much to answer a closed-ended question, asking such questions may not start a discussion. "Juan, what goal have you decided to work on?" would result in more talk. Using open-ended questions will require practice on your part; they usually begin with HOW or WHAT.

Rephrasing or reflecting involves restating in your own words what another person has said. For example, if someone says, "I'd like to go out for the band, but I'm afraid I won't make the team," you might say, "You don't want to go out for the band because you don't think you are good enough." Rephrasing or reflecting a comment helps discussion by showing that you understand. In addition, it enables you to focus on the most important part of the comment.

Including personal examples encourages youth to talk about themselves and their own personal examples. Not only will they feel more comfortable sharing their own examples, but hearing about your story will give them a model of what and how they should share. For example, if you tell them the difficulties you are having in reaching your goals, they may feel more comfortable in talking about their difficulties. Albert Einstein once said: "Setting an example is not the main means of influencing others, it is the only means."

Because learning to lead discussions effectively is a skill and takes practice to do it well, you will need to practice these skills on your own.

How to Manage a Group

If you are working with a group of youth and you do not have much experience, the following are a few tips for success.

Gain Your Group's Respect, Not Their Friendship

Managing a group means keeping everyone focused on what you are teaching. To be an effective leader requires that you develop a certain attitude—this attitude relates to respect. As a leader you have a unique and difficult role. You are not a teacher and not a friend; you are somewhere in between. The key to this role is *respect*—the group's respect for you and your respect for them. Think of someone you respect and how that person earned your respect. Probably they have some of the following qualities.

- Lead by example
- Predictable and consistent
- Fair and trustworthy
- Give you honest feedback
- Care about you without being your pal
- Show you respect

Whenever you are trying to establish a leadership role, it is easier to develop and maintain a respectful and productive atmosphere by being stricter early on. If the group respects you in the beginning and understand how they are supposed to relate to you, a positive atmosphere has been created and most likely will be maintained. If you try to become stricter as you go on, you will very likely be fighting an uphill, losing battle.

Create a Positive Learning Environment

You are managing the group so they can learn the life skills being taught. We have developed some rules to help you create an environment where everyone can learn and have fun. These rules are:

Rule 1: Everyone participates.

Rule 2: Everyone must respect and support each other.

It is up to you to enforce the rules and to keep the group focused on what you are teaching.

Problems You May Encounter in Managing Your Group

Youth are often easily distracted. Some will want to speak more than others, and some may not want to speak at all. Try not to let one or two dominate. Encourage everyone to participate in the discussion and activities. For example, to get more discussion from the group you might say, "We haven't heard from everybody; what are some other ideas?"

If someone is very quiet, you can draw him or her into the discussion by asking an open-ended question. A question such as "Crystal, how do you feel about that?" lets her know that you are interested in what she has to say. It is important not to embarrass anyone. If a person does not want to talk, that is OK. As they feel more comfortable they will participate more.

When the group gets excited, nervous, or embarrassed, everyone may want to talk at once, and it can become noisy. You will need to control the group by quieting them down when necessary, asking friends not to talk to each other, and reminding them to respect the ideas and comments of others. Keeping control while encouraging discussion is a challenge.

Sometimes some group members will intentionally make comments that don't fit, are inappropriate, or distract the group. Ignore such comments as best as you can. It is important not to let these comments get you off track.

Another way to manage your group is by standing or sitting close to group members who are disruptive. Many individuals who are distracted (for example, whispering, rough-housing, and fiddling with items) need help in focusing on tasks. The less you have to discipline, the better the learning atmosphere. You can also ask group members who are distracting to move to other seats. Many times, nothing more needs to be done.

Nonverbal Communication: You Are What You Do

Nonverbal communication can make or break a workshop. Indeed, some believe that most communication is nonverbal. Think about the meaning of a simple smile or how people raise their voice or pound their fists to emphasize a point. Your nonverbal behavior can provide clues to the group about how you feel. For instance, if you look bored and uninterested, they will quickly become bored and restless. A lively, enthusiastic leader can bring some life to the dullest of groups. The following sections address specific areas of nonverbal communication and provide helpful hints for improving techniques.

The Dos and Don'ts of Eye Contact

DO:

- Look at the group while speaking and look around the room at everyone in attendance.
- Look at people who are not paying attention because this is an effective way to bring them back into the group.

DON'T:

- Stare at the manual, floor, walls, or directly at people while speaking.
- Always look at the people who are paying attention. (This is very tempting because these people will smile, nod, and seem to understand).

Your Body Talks for You

Body movements can be used to emphasize a point; nervous habits can distract the audience and decrease your effectiveness. When you are nervous you tend to fidget, swing your legs, or play with pens and pencils. These behaviors, as well as chewing gum or playing with your hair, are very distracting and should be avoided when you talk or when you are listening. Body movements can encourage involvement. Move around during the session. Walking around the group helps to keep their attention. It's not just what you say but how you say it:

- Talk so that everyone can hear you.
- Maintain an even pace. Avoid talking too fast or too slow.
- Use simple words—not everyone will know all the words you do. Explain any words that are unfamiliar.
- Add some expression to your voice. Avoid speaking in a monotone.
- Avoid saying "you know," "um," or "ah" all the time—it can be very distracting.
- Arrange your space so everyone feels part of the group.

The Importance of Giving Feedback

To learn the skills taught, youth must constantly know how they are doing. This process of providing others information about their skill level is called feedback. A large part of your success in having the group effectively learn life skills is dependent on how well you give feedback. Without constructive feedback, they will not know their weaknesses or their strengths.

Giving effective feedback is a skill. For it to be effective it has to be given so that a person can hear it. Effective feedback is:

- Given as promptly as possible;
- Concise; in other words, it does not contain more detail or information than needed;
- Focused on strengths as well as weaknesses;
- Given in a personal and non-threatening manner, avoiding moral or value judgments;
- Concerned only with behavior the person can control or change;
- Discussed until it is understood; and
- Definite---it is not given and then "taken back."

Examples of ineffective feedback include saying things such as, "I don't like the color of your eyes. It's so distracting." or "Your goal is too weird."

Effective feedback is often given as if it were a sandwich. First, start with something positive about someone's actions. Then, make one constructive comment about what might be improved. Follow up with some suggestions about how to improve and then finish with a positive note. For example, "Sarah that was a really great effort you put forth. Next time I would like you to try stay focused on your follow-through a few seconds longer. You are making good progress, keep up the good work."

Tips for Successful Sessions

Prepare

- Take a few minutes to skim through the relevant life skill session before teaching it. Read over the session all the way through.
- Go over it again, and on a separate piece of paper, write down the main activities. For each activity:
  - Include the purpose for doing the activity
  - Write out the first sentence you will say to introduce the activity
  - Write down a personal example for any activities that require it

Practice

There are several ways to practice and you will find some work better than others for your own preparation. Here are few suggestions:

- Present the session in front of a mirror.
- Pretend to present the session in front of a lot of people.
- Present the session to a friend, a sibling, or a parent.

- Present the session with your eyes closed, imagining you are in the classroom.

Remember
- You do not have to memorize a whole life skills session. Refer to the material when needed.
- Do not be afraid to mess up. It does not have to be perfect.
- Be yourself.

Overview

In this overview we include the overall purpose of each session, as well as all of the materials needed, as this will help for planning. We recommend that you teach all of the life skills in the order they are presented. However, as previously mentioned, we wanted to develop a resource that could be flexible. Therefore, if you do not have the time permitted to teach all of these sessions then you can follow the following recommendations for an adapted version.

- If working with a group of youth, Session 1 should always be the first session taught because this will help foster good teamwork, which is particularly important for new groups but also valuable for existing groups when beginning a new program.
- Goal setting is a skill that takes time to develop and master. It is also the foundational life skill in the larger program we have developed. As a result, it is highly recommended that you complete Session 2–7.
- From the remainder of the sessions you can choose which ones to include based upon the amount of time you have remaining for your specific program/group/team.
- Finally, once the activities of any particular session are complete it is important to debrief the youth about what they have learned and how they can take what they have learned in the session and transfer it to other parts of their life (e.g., school, work, home, peers).

Team Building and Appreciating Differences
Purpose: To help youth get to know one another and appreciate each other
Materials needed: 2 beach balls, a permanent marker

Setting Goals: Part I
Purpose: To help the youth identify their dreams and begin to understand the four components of a reachable goal
Materials needed: Enough 3x5 cards or small pieces of paper for every youth in the group, a target, a ball/object to throw at target, session worksheet(s), and a pen/pencil for each participant

Setting Goals: Part II
Purpose: To help youth continue to learn about the four components of a reachable goal

Materials needed: Blindfolds, 10 sheets of paper/targets that the youth can step on, a small ball with a small box or container that the ball can fit into, and a phone or stop-watch to keep time

Setting Your Goal

Purpose: For youth to learn how to set a reachable goal they want to achieve in two months

Materials needed: Session worksheet(s), and a pen/pencil for each participant

Making a Goal Ladder

Purpose: To understand the importance of developing a plan for the goal they set

Materials needed: White board, chalk board or large post-it paper, session worksheet(s), and a pen/pencil for each participant

Identifying and Overcoming Roadblocks

Purpose: To help youth recognize and overcome potential roadblocks to reaching their goals

Materials needed: Session worksheet(s), and a pen/pencil for each participant

Developing a Social Support Team

Purpose: To help youth identify a social support team that can help them in reaching their goal

Materials needed: Session worksheet(s), and a pen/pencil for each participant

Using Positive Self-Talk

Purpose: To help youth become aware of their own self-talk and make it positive

Materials needed: Session worksheet(s), pen/pencil, beads with letters, and string or bracelets that can be written on

Building Confidence and Courage

Purpose: To help youth develop confidence in themselves

Materials needed: Session worksheet(s) and a pen/pencil for each participant

Maintaining Focus

Purpose: To help youth learn about what focus is and practice their focusing skills

Materials needed: Session worksheet(s), a pen/pencil for each participant, and colored markers

Learning to Relax

Purpose: To help youth learn how they can relax

Materials needed: None

Managing Emotions

Purpose: To help youth to be able to control their emotions in different situations

Materials needed: Session worksheet(s) and a pen/pencil for each participant

Defining and Accepting Responsibility

Purpose: To help youth learn how to take responsibility for their actions

Materials needed: Session worksheet(s) and a pen/pencil for each participant

Respecting Others

Purpose: To help youth learn about the importance of and how to respect others

Materials needed: Balloons, markers, session worksheet(s), and a pen/pencil for each participant

Managing Your Time

Purpose: To help youth learn strategies to manage their time more effectively

Materials needed: Session worksheet(s) and a pen/pencil for each participant

Becoming a Leader

Purpose: To help youth learn about what leadership is and how they may become a leader

Materials needed: Chart paper, markers, session worksheet(s), and a pen/pencil for each participant

Developing a Healthy Lifestyle

Purpose: To help youth learn about how they can incorporate other healthy living practices

Materials needed: Session worksheet(s) and a pen/pencil for each participant

Reviewing Goals and Personal Performance

Purpose: To help youth learn how to adjust goals as well as celebrate goals achieved

Materials needed: Session worksheet(s) and a pen/pencil for each participant

Team Building and Appreciating Differences

Team building is a process of bringing a group of individuals together to foster positive relationships and work on a shared goal. Appreciating differences is part of the team-building process and occurs when everyone in the group can appreciate the strengths that each individual can bring to the group, and is also aware of each individual's areas for improvement.

Given that this is the first session of the program and may be the first time this group has met, it is important to spend a few minutes introducing yourself and going over some of the basic ground rules.

Introduction and Rules (5 Minutes)

Introduce yourself as the leader of the group. Make sure your introduction enables the group to identify with you as much as possible. For example, you might include: your name and nickname, your position, what you do outside of the program (e.g., work, school), your favorite sport or activity in which you participate, and why you wanted to be a leader for this program.

Next give an overview of the program. At this point it will be important to explain what life skills are. You can start this conversation by asking the youth what they think the term _life skills_ means. If they have trouble, ask them what kinds of skills they think they need to succeed in life. Finally, it may be helpful to choose a name for your group or team if they do not already have one. Try to avoid a name that is the same as a local team. Be creative.

Team Building Activities (10–15 Minutes)

Play one or both of the name game activities described in the following sections to help you and your group get to know each other better. Option 1A and 1B are for new groups in which the group members have not previously met, while Option 2 is typically used when the members know each other by name but are still getting to know one another.

Option 1A: Hot Ball Name

For this activity you need some type of ball (it can even be paper wrapped as a ball) that is easy for the group members to catch.

1. Have everyone gather into a circle.
2. Explain that this game is a lot like hot potato. Each person tosses the ball to a different person in the circle, as if the ball is too hot to hold for very long.
3. When the ball is tossed to a person for the first time, toss and catch it long enough to say his or her name and nickname and then toss it to someone else.
4. After the ball has been passed to participants twice, go around again and have the thrower name the receiver before tossing the ball.

Option 1B: Names in Motion

1. Have everyone gather into a circle.
2. Explain that this game is called Names in Motion because you have to introduce yourself by taking one step forward into the circle, say your name, and do some motion. (Note: The motion can be anything from a wave, to a jumping jack, to a few dance steps. Encourage creativity and originality).
3. After each person introduces himself or herself with their motion and steps back into the circle, the other people in the circle take one step forward and repeat the person's name and motion. Everyone then steps back into the circle and the next person introduces himself or herself.

Option 2: Beach Ball Bonanza

For this activity you will need a beach ball and a permanent marker (if you have a large group you should have one ball for every 10–15 people). Once you have these materials, blow up the beach ball and with the permanent marker write down "get to know you" questions all over the ball. Following is a list of possible questions. Feel free to also use any questions that you believe would be good for the specific group with which you are working. Choose the questions most appropriate for the ages of the group.

- Where were you born?
- What is your favorite super hero?
- Chocolate or vanilla?
- Where do you want to go for your next vacation?
- Favorite food?
- What would you do with $1,000,000?
- When is your birthday?
- Favorite movie or TV show?
- Do you have siblings?
- Favorite color?
- Favorite animal?

- Would you live on Mars?
- Favorite subject in school?
- Favorite physical activity or sport?
- What do you want to be when you grow up?
- What are you afraid of?

Once you have written the questions on the ball you are ready to start the activity.

- Have the group gather into a circle.
- Hand one person the beach ball. Have him or her read aloud the question closest to his or her right thumb and answer the question.
- Once the question is answered, the person then throws the ball to someone in the circle. The person who catches the ball reads aloud the question closest to his or her right thumb and answers the question.
- Continue to have the group members share with each other until everyone has had at least two turns.
- If you have a large group that you have broken into multiple groups, have each group allow everyone to respond to a question at least once and then switch the groups and continue.

Appreciating Differences (10–15 Minutes)

Appreciating differences is an important component of the team-building process. Being able to appreciate differences is also very important when working with a group to help them recognize that everyone in the group has a particular function or role and to understand what that particular role or function is. If the group members can appreciate one another's differences and how these differences lead to the various group members having different but important contributions to the group, the group is more likely to function effectively.

Following are a few activities that you can do with groups to help them begin to understand how to appreciate differences and to understand that in many cases the differences do not matter. Start with Activity 1.1. If you have time, as well as a more mature group, you can also complete Activity 1.2.

Activity 1.1 Differences – What Matters?

Have the group come together and explain that you are going to give a series of directions and that they should either make their way left or right depending on their response. After each direction have them look around to see who is in their group, observing who is similar to them and who is different than them. Then have them come back to the center and repeat this process for each direction.

Directions:

- Go left if you like to sleep late; if not, go right
- Go left if you identify as male; if not, go right
- Go left if you like desserts; if not, go right
- Go left if you are older than 25; if not, go right (state whatever age will separate the group)
- Go left if you like scary movies; if not, go right
- Go left if you have a nickname you use; if not, go right
- Go left if you have more than one sibling; if not, go right
- Go left if you like to cuddle; if not, go right
- Go left if you want to be rich; if not, go right
- Go left if you want to be famous; if not, go right

Bring the group back together (they can sit down for this if they want) to disciss:

- Were you surprised about who was in or not in your group for any of the directions?
- Can you think of a situation in which any of these differences would be important for achieving your group or team goal?
- If not, what characteristics are important to help achieve the group's goal? (Below are some you can share to get the group thinking—use those most relevant to the group.)
  - To keep cool under pressure
  - To be strong
  - To problem solve
  - To manage others
  - To be able to share
  - To help others
  - To make everyone laugh
  - To stay focused
  - To persevere
  - To be creative
  - To be able to write
  - To lead
  - To follow instructions

Then ask the group the following questions:

- Were these differences more important than the first one discussed?
- If so, why are some differences more important than others?
- How do we determine what differences are important?

You can help focus the discussion on the idea that usually it is not the physical characteristics or personal preferences that are important for working together, it is rather the variety of skills that each person brings to the group. Although everyone might not share the same interests, everyone has different strengths they can bring to the group. You can share with the group that in life, we benefit from teaming up with people who have different skills—people with different ways of dealing with challenges or with skills in areas in which we are not as strong. They can help us see and learn.

Activity 1.2 Bringing Together the Best of Everyone

1. Have everyone gather and sit in a circle.
2. Explain that this is an activity to help each other learn about the strengths and areas of improvement for each member of the group.
3. Ask for a volunteer to start by stating a strength they possess to help the group achieve the group goal, as well as an area they would like to develop.
4. Continue around the circle so that everyone has a chance to share, but explain to the group that each person should identify a different strength—it can be similar to someone else's but should be unique to what they can bring to the group.
5. As you complete the activity tell the group that they should pay attention to who they believe in the group could help them with something they need to improve based on the strengths shared.
6. Once everyone has shared their strengths and areas of development discuss how the group members can help each other—how they can match strengths with areas of development.

Debrief and Transfer (5 Minutes)

Once you have completed the activities it is recommended to have the group debrief their experiences with the activities and talk about how to transfer what they have learned to other domains in their lives. You may want to ask the following questions:

- What life skill did you learn about today?
- What does team building or teamwork mean to you?
- What does it mean to appreciate differences in others?
- What might you share with others about what you have learned?
- How can you work with others at school? Home?
- How can you help your peers or family members feel appreciated for their unique strengths?

Setting Goals: Part A

Only you can keep yourself from reaching your dreams. — *Henry David Thoreau*

The Importance of Dreams (5 Minutes)

Ask the youth or group, "What is a dream?" The most likely responses may be that dreams are things that occur while sleeping or they are things that we want in the future. It is important to differentiate between a dream we have in our sleep and a dream we have for our future. You can explain that dreams—at least the ones they will be thinking about today—are their future dreams—what they want for themselves when they are older. They can have more than one dream for their future. Also encourage them to dream big and not put any limits on their dreams. You can then explain that they will now participate in some activities that will represent the first step in reaching their dreams.

Trip to the Future (10 Minutes)

Tell members of the group to imagine adding 10 years to their current age. Ask them who they know who is that age now (this will provide a reference point for them). Then tell them:

> "Dreams are what you want for yourself. You can have many different dreams. Think of some of the dreams you have for your future. Think of your best possible future—the things you would most like to happen."

As a leader of the group, share some of your dreams in these areas (e.g., "When I was your age, my dreams were …"). You are role models, so it is important that you share your experiences as much as possible.

Have the group write down their dreams in the worksheet Destination: My Future worksheet. Encourage them to right down their best possible dreams—the things they would most like to happen. Then share with the group some of their dreams.

Destination: My Future

Ten years from now I will be _____ years old.

What am I good at?

_____

_____

What am I interested in?

_____

_____

What would I like to be doing in 10 years?

_____

_____

What do I want my life to be like in 10 years?

_____

_____

Turning Dreams into Goals (5 Minutes)

Ask the group why goals are important and how they can help us. If participants are having trouble thinking of ways, here are some tips.

- Give participants motivation.
- Help participants to make plans for the future.
- Give participants direction.
- Give participants a sense of success and pride in our accomplishments.

Making Your Goal Reachable (20 Minutes)

The purpose of this set of activities is to help youth understand that the way they set their goals affects whether they reach them.

Tell the group there are four steps to making goals reachable. Goals must be important to you, stated positively, specific, and under your control. Activities in this session deal with the first two aspects—important and positively stated goals. Session Three address how to make goals specific and under your control.

Goals Must Be Important to You
Trading a Dream (10 Minutes)

Have the youth write a non-sport or non-activity dream that is important to them.

1. On a 3x5 card. If working with a group, collect the cards, shuffle them, and have them choose a new card without looking at it. If working with an individual youth, write your own dream on a 3x5 card and then exchange cards with the youth.

2. Allow a minute or so to think about the new dream on the card and ask them the following four questions:

- What is it like to have someone else's goal?
- Do you think that this goalwould be important to you?
- Do you think that you would be willing to work as hard for the goal that was given to you, or do you think that you would work harder for the goal that you came up with on your own?
- If the goal was not important to anyone else (e.g., parents, coaches, friends), would it still be important to you?

Goals Must Be Stated Positively
The Positive Game (10–15 Minutes)

The purpose of this activity is to demonstrate to participants that energy follows attention. The participants will make a positive or negative statement to themselves and then attempt to hit a target with an object specific to the chosen sport or activity.

1. Set up a target specific to their sport or activity; if a target does not exist in their sport pick a sport or activity with which the group is familiar.

2. Select two volunteers with different skill levels to participate in this activity. Have each volunteer complete both activities, one at a time. Have the first volunteer stand a challenging distance from the target. Note: Choose a distance so that the average participant should be able to hit the target 50 % of the time.

3. Explain that the volunteer will have five attempts to hit the target. Before each attempt, the volunteer must repeat the words, "I don't want to miss," three to five times.

4. Now have the same volunteer repeat the exercise, but say instead: "I will hit the target" three to five times before each of five attempts. Note: You may modify this statement to a more sport-specific positive statement. Count how many attempts hit the target.

Talk with the group about their reactions to what they just experienced. You may want to ask them the differences between what they said for the first five attempts, and what they said for the next five attempts. Emphasize that the statement for the first five attempts was more negative; it was telling them what they should *not* do rather that what they should do. Then ask them how they felt when they took the first five shots compared to the next five shots. Reinforce statements when they say that they felt more confident, more relaxed, and less nervous when they took the second five shots. Then explain that, when we state something positively, we create a picture in our mind of what it is we want to have happen, rather than something we don't want to have happen. Your body will listen to what you tell it to do. Positively stated goals never have words like cannot, not, or avoid in them.

Debrief and Transfer (5 minutes)

Once you have completed the activities it is good to debrief their experiences with the activities and to talk about how to transfer what they have learned to other domains in their lives. You may want to ask the following questions:

- What life skill did you learn about today?
- Why is setting goals important?
- What are the four characteristics of reaching a goal?
- Why is it important to have a goal that is important to you?
- What goals can you set for yourself at school, home?

Setting Goals: Part B

If you aim at nothing you will hit it every time. — Unknown

Review (5 minutes)

In the last session, we learned that the first two characteristics of a reachable goal are: important to you and stated positively. Then explain that in today's session they will learn about: making their goal specific and under their control.

Goals Must Be Specific

If a goal is too general or not specific, it is difficult to know when it has been achieved. Goals that are not specific enough often have words like *good*, *better*, *more*, and *less* in them.

The following activity will help reinforce the importance of having specific direction when you want to go somewhere, just like your goal needs to be specific to reach it. If you are working with a youth one-on-one you can adapt the activity so that the youth is blindfolded and you are the one providing direction and you can also do the reverse to help reinforce the importance of being specific.

Activity 3.1 Blindfolded Relay Race (10–15 Minutes)

This activity can be done in a large room or outside.

1. Choose one or two volunteers who have not already participated in an activity.
2. For each youth place 10 sheets of paper/targets in a random zigzag fashion but make sure to have a start line and a finish line.
3. Blindfold the youth (if you do not have a blindfold have them close their eyes).
4. Explain to the youth that the purpose is to get from the start to the finish line as quickly as possible, making sure to step on each piece of paper/target. Repeat this process twice with the youth and time each one. The first time

give some direction but not too specific (e.g., go forward more, stop, turn around, move again). The second time, to provide very specific directions (e.g., move two steps forward, turn to your right, walk three steps).

When the activity is completed, ask the group what made it difficult or easy to be guided to the finish line. Emphasize that the more specific the directions, the easier it seemed for people to go through the race.

Goals Must Be Under Your Control

Explain to the youth or group that you can only reach goals you control. If the goal requires another person doing something, you cannot be sure the goal will be reached. Following is an activity that can be used to demonstrate how easy control can be taken away when a focus is placed on an outcome rather than the process.

Activity 3.2 How Much of Your Performance Do You Control (10–15 Minutes)

1. Introduce a task that is fairly easy to do. In an office it could be to walk from one wall to another; at the house it could be walking up and down stairs. If you have a ball of any type, ask the youth throw it up in the air and catch it or bounce it. Have them tell you how many times they can complete the task in a minute. Time it and count.

2. Then have the youth repeat the activity, but this time introduce an obstacle (e.g., stand in their way while they are trying to get from one wall to the other or grab their ball; other options are to yell or cheer, have them stand on one foot, tell a joke, try the skill blindfolded—anything to distract the participant). Again, time it for a minute and count.

Once this is complete, discuss with the youth how distractions and obstacles in second activity affected their ability to complete the task as effectively. You can enhance the discussion by asking whether their goal for the task (how many times per minute) was within their control. Discuss what was in their control. Then talk about other kinds of things in their environment that are in their control. Explain that you can only reach goals that are a result of your actions, from things that are under your control. If the goal requires another person being involved, you cannot be sure the goal will be reached.

Debrief and Transfer (5 Minutes)

Once you have completed the activities it is recommended to have the group debrief their experiences with the activities and to talk about how they can transfer what they have learned to other domains in their lives. You may want to ask the following questions:

- What characteristics of a goal did youth learn about today?
- What does "under your control" mean?
- How can you be more specific with goals you have for school?
- How can you ensure that your goals outside of this program are under your control?

Setting Your Goal

A person without a goal is like a computer without a program. — Steve Danish

Review (5 Minutes)

Remind the youth or group of the four characteristics of a reachable goal that were discussed in Session 2 and Session 3. Goals must be 1) important to you, 2) stated positively, 3) specific, and 4) under your control. In this session the youth will set a two-month goal for themselves. If you are working one-on-one or with a small group (i.e., less than five) it is possible to combine this session and the next (making a goal ladder) into one. However, with large groups more time is needed to oversee their goals in some capacity to ensure that they are written effectively.

Setting a Life Goal (30 Minutes)

Ask the youth or group to write down on their Setting Goals Worksheet (on page 111) a goal that they want to achieve in the next 6–8 weeks. You as the leader should also have a goal so that you can provide the participants with an example and also to show them that you are working towards a goal.

My Goal

In this session the participants will spend the majority of the time setting one goal. It is your responsibility to assist the participants so that everyone sets a goal that is stated positively, specific, important to them, and under their control. It may be effective for participants to spend 5–10 minutes doing the best that they can and then have them engage in a cooperative game or activity while you work one-on-one (calling each person over and reviewing their goal with them).

Review their goals individually using the questions that follow as a guide.

Important to You

1. Do they know how reaching this goal will help them be closer to their dream?

2. Can they see themselves working hard to reach this goal?
3. Can they describe how they will feel if they reach this goal?

Stated Positively

1. What picture do they have of this goal? Do they see exactly what action they want to take?
2. Have words such as *not*, *stop*, *avoid*, or *don't* been used? These words make the goal negatively rather that positively stated.

Stated Specifically

1. Is it clear to them (and you) when they will have reached the goal? What types of things will happen?
2. Have words like *more*, *less*, or *better* been used? These words make the goal statement not specific.

Under Your Control

1. Are they most responsible for making this happen? Are there others involved in evaluating or determining if this goal is reached (e.g., coach giving more playing time, teacher grading an exam/assignment)?
2. Can the goal be achieved during the next 6–8 weeks?

Debrief and Transfer (5 Minutes)

Once you have completed the activities it is recommended to have the group debrief their experiences with the activities and to talk about how they can transfer what they have learned to other domains in their lives. You may want to ask the following questions:

- What did you learn about writing out a goal?
- Is it difficult to make a goal meet the four characteristics of a reachable goal? In what ways?
- What other goals do you have for school, home, or a sport that you can write down?

Setting Goals Worksheet

Write down a goal you want to reach in 6–8 weeks.

_____

_____

_____

_____

_____

_____

_____

For a goal to be reachable it must have four characteristics:

1. important to you,
2. stated positively,
3. specific, and
4. under your control.

Remember, positively stated goals never have words like *cannot*, *not*, or *avoid* in them. Goals that are not specific enough often have words like *good*, *better*, *more*, and *less* in them. Finally, if the goal requires another person doing something, you cannot be sure the goal will be reached. Ask yourself, "Am I able to reach this goal by doing something myself?"

Notes

Making a Goal Ladder

If you have built castles in the air, your work need not be lost; that is where they should be. Now put foundations under them. — *Henry David Thoreau*

Review (5 Minutes)

Remind the group that there are four characteristics of a reachable goal. Goals must be 1) important to you, 2) stated positively, 3) specific, and 4) under your control.

Activity 5.1 Making a Goal Ladder (15 Minutes)

Explain to the youth/group that the first step in reaching any goal is to make a plan. This plan is what we call a goal ladder. Once you have established a goal ladder, you work your way up the ladder, one step at a time. The goal ladder is important because it helps to break down goals into small, reachable steps. A goal ladder also helps participants to see their progress toward their goal.

Have the youth or group work with one of your goals and help you make a goal ladder. The rationale for this is that if you can work through one together, they will learn how as well as increase their confidence for developing their own goal ladder.

1. Think of all the things you can do right now to reach your goal. Have the youth write these down on a white board, chalk board, or large post-it paper. You want to have at least six steps.

2. Go through each step together and determine whether that step is truly a necessity to have on your goal ladder.

3. Make sure that each step on the ladder is positively stated, specific, and under your control. Rewrite them when necessary.

4. Next, put the steps in order based on what you should do first, second, third, etc. Make sure to have at least six rungs on your ladder.

Activity 5.2 Making an Individual Goal Ladder (15 Minutes)

Now that the youth have assisted you in creating a goal ladder for one of your goals, have them develop a goal ladder for their own goal. Have them use the Goal Ladder Worksheet to help them complete a goal ladder for their goal.

Debrief and Transfer (5 Minutes)

Once you have completed the activities it is good to have the group debrief their experiences with the activities and to talk about how they can transfer what they have learned to other domains in their lives. You may want to ask the following questions:

- What is the purpose of creating a goal ladder?
- How can it help you reach your goal?
- Can a goal ladder help you reach your other goals?
- What goal ladder will you create next?

Goal Ladder Worksheet

Step 1: Write the goal that you have set (remember it should be a goal to reach in 6–8 weeks and it should be positive, specific, important to you, and under your control).

Goal:_____

_____

_____

_____

Step 2: In the space below, list or draw everything you must do to reach your goal. Try to have at least 6, but more likely, 8–10 things you need to do to achieve your goal.

_____

Step 3: Take all of the things you put in Step 2 and write them out using the characteristics of a reachable goal (i.e., positive, specific, important to you, and under your control).

- _____
  _____

- _____
  _____

- _____
  _____

- _____
  _____

- _____
  _____

- _____
  _____

- _____
  _____

- _____
  _____

- _____
  _____

- _____
  _____

Step 4: Put a #1 next to the item you expect to do first, a #2 next to the item you expect to do second, and so on. As you do this activity the first step should be one that is fairly easy to accomplish.

Step 5: Using your order, fill in the goal ladder on the next page step by step. Make sure step #1 is on the bottom rung (just like a real ladder). For examples, in step #1 (at the bottom) write what you expect to do first, in step #2 write what you expect to do second, and so on. Then write a target date when you expect to complete each step.

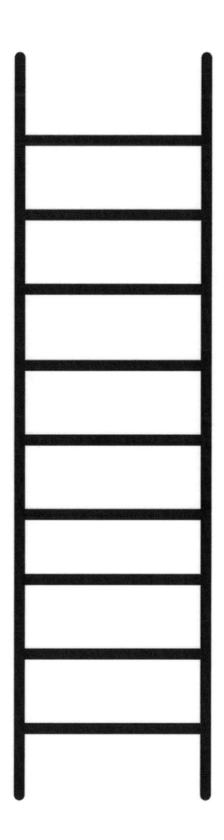

Notes

Identifying and Overcoming Roadblocks

If you find a path with no obstacles, it probably doesn't lead anywhere. — Unknown

Identifying Roadblocks (20 Minutes)

To start the session off it is recommended to ask the group to think about what a roadblock is and how that might relate to achieving their goal. Ask the group to give examples of traffic roadblocks. Examples might include fallen trees, street construction, traffic accidents, and police barricades. Explain the connection between traffic roadblocks and roadblocks to reaching your goals—both get in the way of their desired destination. A roadblock is something that prevents them from reaching your goal.

Once the youth have a good understanding of what a roadblock is, you can help them understand the three common types of roadblocks by using the following examples.

Lack of Knowledge

This happens when you do not have all the information needed to reach all the steps in the goal ladder (e.g., if your goal is to complete a big school project but you do not know where to find the information you need to start working on it).

Lack of Skill

This happens when you do not know how to do something that is important for reaching your goal (e.g., if you are involved in a sport and your goal is to complete a particular routine or run a farther distance but you do not have all of the skills to reach that goal).

Lack of Social Support

This happens when you need the support or help of others to achieve your goal (e.g., if you have a school project and you need supplies, you would need support or help from your parents, teachers, or older siblings to get those supplies for you).

You should explain to the youth that roadblocks could also be things such as

- not working hard or giving up on yourself;
- engaging in health-compromising behaviors (e.g., drugs, alcohol, tobacco);
- injury;
- not taking care of yourself (e.g., not eating healthy or getting enough sleep); and
- not having enough confidence.

You can use the Identifying Roadblocks Worksheet on the next page to help youth identify their own potential roadblocks. This can be used when working one-on-one or in small groups. However, remember the younger the youth are, the more help they are going to need to figure out what some roadblocks might be and how they can overcome them.

Overcoming Roadblocks (10 Minutes)

There is a short acronym we developed that you can teach youth to help them learn how to problem solve to overcome the roadblocks they may face when trying to reach their goals. There are four steps in this problem-solving strategy: S – stop, T – think, A – anticipate, R – respond.

S stands for *stop* and take a deep breath. When you feel a lot of pressure or feel frustrated when faced with a potential roadblock it helps to take a deep breath. You could ask the youth how doing that would calm them down, and what other things they can do to calm down or relieve pressure or frustration.

T stands for *think* of all your choices. For example, think of the type of roadblock you have and what you can do, or who you can seek help from, to overcome the roadblock. You may also be in a situation in which you have different choices, some of which will help you reach your goal, but others might not. For example, a friend of yours may want you to do something that might prevent you from reaching your goal or dream. Ask your group the following questions:

- What roadblock are you facing?
- What are some of the choices you have in this situation?
- Who or what can help you?

A stands for *anticipate* the consequences of each choice. Anticipate means to look ahead. A consequence is what happens as a result of something else, and consequences can be good or bad. You can ask the youth how their choices will affect their ability to reach their goals, and what are some consequences they may face from their choices.

R stands for *respond* with the best choice. Youth should always ask themselves what is the best choice for them, and how can they make that choice.
Try to reinforce that the best choice is the one that move towards achieving their goal. The second worksheet at the end of this section will allow the youth to plan out each of

the steps to overcome a potential roadblock they may face.

Debrief and Transfer (5 Minutes)

Once you have completed the activities it is recommended to have the group debrief their experiences with the activities and to talk about how they can transfer what they have learned to other domains in their lives. You may want to ask the following questions:

- What is a roadblock?
- What roadblocks have you or will you face outside of this program/session?
- What did you learn today that can help you at school, home, work, or with friends?

Identifying Roadblocks Worksheet

Knowledge	Skills	Social Support
What do I need to know?	**What skills do I need?**	**Who do I need to help me?**
Where can I find this information?	**How can I learn them?**	**How can they help me?**

Take a deep breath
Think about all the choices you have for the decision you have to make.

1._____

_____

2._____

_____

3._____

_____

Anticipate all of the consequences of each choice.

Choice 1	Choice 2	Choice 3

Respond with the best choice.

Notes

Developing a Social Support Team

No one is an island. Everyone is part of the world. — Adapted from John Donne

Circle of Support (10 Minutes)

Explain to the group that sometimes reaching our goals and making good decisions involves getting help or support from others. It does not mean they do the work for us, but they can support and mentor us along the way. The following activity, Circle of Support, is designed for a group. However, you can do a similar activity if working one-on-one with a youth.

One-on-One

Have the youth stand up and get into a position where he or she is pretending to sit on chair (like a squat) and hold it for a few seconds. It will likely be difficult as it involves balance and no support. Have the youth rest and now stand back to back with you and squat together, leaning on each other for support. Talk to the youth about how when the two of you did the activity together, leaning on each other, it was easier to do. This activity is a great example of why getting support from others is often helpful.

Group Activity

To make it work, everyone in the circle must support everyone else. Make sure that the end product is a tight circle made up of people sitting on the knees of the person behind them with the person in front of them on their knees. As you do the activity, state each of the steps one at a time. Wait until the entire group has completed each step before proceeding to the next step.

1: Everyone stand up and get into a large circle.
2: Make sure that the tallest person is not next to the shortest person – if so rearrange.
Step 3: Hold hands with the two people next to you.
Step 4: Make sure the circle is perfectly round, so adjust as needed.

5: Take one regular step into the center.

6: Make sure the circle is perfectly round again, so adjust as needed.

7: Now, take another step into the center. (Repeat Steps 6 and 7 until everyone is standing shoulder to shoulder in a perfect circle.)

8: Let go of the hands of the people next to you.

9: Everyone turn to your left, putting your right hip in toward the center.

10: Look down at your feet. Move toward the center so that the toe of your right foot is almost touching the heel of the right foot of the person in front of you.

11: Lightly place your hands on the shoulders of the person in front you.

12: At the count of three, slowly sit on the knees of the person behind you.

13: Remember, if one of us falls, we *all* fall.

14: 1-2-3, slowly sit down. (Keep trying until your group is successful.)

15: Let's see if we can hold this for five seconds and then slowly stand up. Count together. 1-2-3-4-5, stand up!

Goal Keepers and Goal Busters (10 Minutes)

Explain to the youth or group that there are people in our lives who can support us and help us achieve our goals. These people are called goal keepers. For example, a coach may help you by teaching you a new skill or your teammates may help you by cheering for you when you are playing or competing. Also explain that there are also people who try to get in the way or prevent you from reaching your goals. These people are called goal busters. For example, a goal buster might try and get you to stay out late the night before you have a big game or to use drugs or alcohol. Also, a goal buster is any person who tells you that you won't reach your goal. It is important that you choose to be surrounded by goal keepers to help you reach your goal and to stay away from goal busters who will only get in the way of your success.

Creating a Dream Team (15 Minutes)

Have the group create their own "dream team" on the worksheet at the end of this section. Explain that there may be different dream team members but that there are important characteristics of a good dream team. Your dream team should be people:

- you see often
- who know your capabilities and your limitations
- who are concerned about you
- you can depend on
- you can help at another time

Ask your group to choose their dream team members. In addition to the characteristics above include family members or others who provide love, support, and caring and will help you reach your dreams and goals when you face roadblocks; include best friends, people who you really trust, and/or people with whom you spend a lot of time; and adults or other people who are older than you that help you and serve as good role models. They may be teachers, coaches, ministers, youth group leaders, and family friends.

When they have identified their dream team members, put a heart by dream team members who provide caring help such as listening and providing encouragement and put a star by dream team members who provide doing help such as taking them places or helping with homework. Explain that some dream team members probably can help in both ways, while others can provide only one type of help. Make sure that the dream team can provide both kinds of help.

If you have time you can have them complete the second worksheet, which involves having the youth write down what they would say or ask their different dream team members to help them.

Once you have completed the activities it is recommended to have the group debrief their experiences with the activities and to talk about how they can transfer what they have learned to other domains in their lives. You may want to ask the following questions:

- What did you learn about today?
- Why is it important to have our own dream teams?
- Can you create a dream team for other areas of your life (e.g., school, sport, work)?
- Who is on this new dream team?

My Dream Team

Star = Doing
Heart = Caring

Name:_____

Name:_____

Name:_____

Name:_____

Name:_____

Name:_____

Write down what you could say to each person to ask what you need them to help you with. Write the exact words you will use so you can practice.

_____
_____
_____
_____
_____
_____
_____
_____
_____
_____
_____
_____
_____
_____
_____
_____
_____
_____
_____
_____

Using Positive Self-Talk

When you doubt yourself it is like joining your enemy's army and bearing arms against yourself. You make your failure certain by being the first person to be convinced of it. — *Adapted from Alexandre Dumas*

Listening to What You Say (15 Minutes)

Explain to the youth or group of youth that self-talk is what you think and say to yourself. The way you talk to yourself impacts how you behave, how you communicate, and how you perform, but you may not even realize that you are telling yourself to focus on failure, negative events, and negative feelings. You can help youth become more aware of their own self-talk by using the following questions or discussion points.

1. Listen to what you are telling yourself.
2. What do you usually say to yourself if you answer a question wrong or perform poorly in a competition or on a test? Is it negative or positive?
3. Would you say the same thing to a friend that you say to yourself or let a friend say that to you? Why not?
4. If what they are saying to themselves is negative, it is important to work on changing those thoughts from negative to positive.

Have the youth complete the first worksheet at the end of this session to become more aware of how participants typically talk to themselves.

Developing Your Power Statements (15 Minutes)

An important part of developing positive self-talk is creating personalized statements that can be used to replace negative thoughts. It is important that these statements be meaningful to them, as this will help participants in reaching their goals. Have the youth develop their own power statements and if there is time ask them to share their power statements with others. You may even reinforce that if they feel nervous about sharing, remind your group that this is the time to start practicing a power statement (I can do this!).

Debrief and Transfer (5 Minutes)

Once you have completed the activities it is recommended to have the group debrief their experiences with the activities and to talk about how they can transfer what they have learned to other domains in their lives. You may want to ask the following questions:

- What is positive self-talk?
- Is there a difference in how you feel when you talk negatively vs. positively to yourself?
- Do you use negative self-statements outside of the program/session (e.g., school, with friends, at work, at home)?
- How can you change your negative thoughts to positive thoughts after you leave here?

Self-Talk Awareness Worksheet

What I tell myself when I am preparing for something important:

_____

_____

_____

What I tell myself when I have done well:

_____

_____

_____

What I tell myself when I have done poorly:

_____

_____

_____

What I usually think about my performance after an important event or competition:

_____

_____

_____

Power Statements Worksheet

Write out your POWER statements in the box below that will help you think positively.

1. _____
   _____
   _____
   _____
   _____

2. _____
   _____
   _____
   _____
   _____

3. _____
   _____
   _____
   _____
   _____

4. _____
   _____
   _____
   _____
   _____

5. _____
   _____
   _____
   _____
   _____

Building Confidence and Courage

Confidence demands a great deal of strength—a strong and determined will; it is marked by a sure and persistent belief in oneself and one's true skill. Believe in your ability; be determined to play your role; allow nothing or no one to come between you and your reachable goal.

— Sherman Curl

Believing in Yourself (10 Minutes)

Explain to the youth or group that confidence is the belief that you can successfully do something. Therefore, having confidence in yourself means believing in yourself. People who believe in themselves: approach new situations positively, are not afraid to fail, learn from their mistakes, have realistic expectations, and are not afraid to ask for help. Have the group complete the What's Great About Me worksheet activity that appears at the end of this session.

Introducing Yourself (10 Minutes)

Explain that when you encounter new people, you should introduce yourself. Ask the group to practive introducing themselves to each other. If working one-on-one, ask the youth introduce themselves to you. Explain that to develop confidence in themselves and in interacting with others they should look at the other person—making eye contact is very important—and speak clearly and loudly enough so the other person can understand them.

Building Confidence (10 Minutes)

Explain to the youth that there are actions you can take to increase your confidence. Some of these include: setting goals; practicing skills you want to improve; getting feedback from coaches, teachers, friends, and family; and using people who can do these skills better than you can as models.

You can also explain that by making ourselves act confidently we can increase our confidence. Ask the youth to participate in the following activity (this can be done individually or in a group) to help them practice acting confidently.

1. Think of a person they know, a superhero or an animal that they think is courageous and confident.
2. Ask everyone to stand up. Once they are all standing, have everyone close their eyes and take a deep breath. Have them act out the person, superhero or animal they are thinking about.
3. Try to imagine how that person, superhero or animal feels like and how they might show that they are courageous and confident.

Sometimes believing in yourself will make difficult situations appear easier. If you believe in yourself others will believe in you too!

Debrief and Transfer (5 Minutes)

Once you have completed the activities it is recommended to have the group debrief their experiences with the activities and to talk about how they can transfer what they have learned to other domains in their lives. You may want to ask the following questions:

- What is confidence?
- Where and how are you confident in yourself at school, home, work, and friends?
- How can the actions you have shown help you feel more confident in school, work, or with friends?

What Is Great About Me?

Think about what you like about yourself. Read the words from Textbok 8.1 and circle the ones that describe you. Circle as many words as you want and add your own words if you feel some are missing.

_____

_____

_____

_____

_____

_____

Textbox 8.1 What is Great About Me

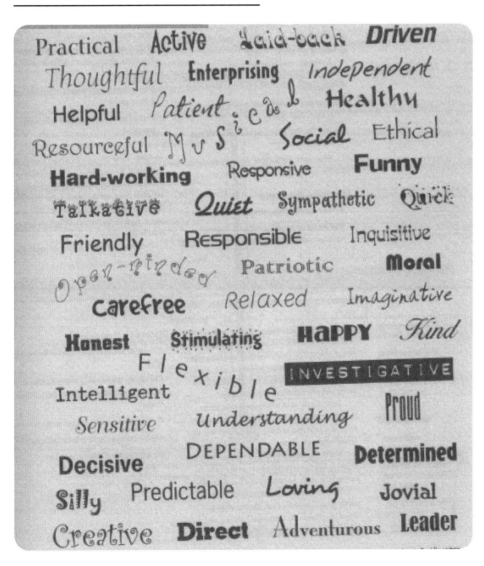

Practical Active Laid-back Driven
Thoughtful Enterprising Independent
Helpful Patient Musical Healthy
Resourceful Musi Social Ethical
Hard-working Responsive Funny
Talkative Quiet Sympathetic Quick
Friendly Responsible Inquisitive
Open-minded Patriotic Moral
Carefree Relaxed Imaginative
Honest Stimulating Happy Kind
Flexible INVESTIGATIVE
Intelligent Proud
Sensitive Understanding
Decisive DEPENDABLE Determined
Silly Predictable Loving Jovial
Creative Direct Adventurous Leader

Notes

Maintaining Focus

"Your focus determines your reality." — *George Lucas*

What Is Focus? (10 Minutes)

Ask the youth or group what the word focus means to them. If they are having difficulty, you can explain that focus is the ability to attend to the important things around them. You can even share the following example.

A student in math class — a subject she typically struggles in — approaches the class ready to focus today. When she sits at her desk, she clears it of anything that she doesn't need, so not to distract her. She keeps her pencil in her hand and her eyes between the chalkboard and her book. Keeping her hands and eyes busy with what she should be doing will help to keep her on task and avoid distractions. When she finds herself getting antsy, she stretches her legs quietly at her desk.

Ask the youth to give examples of when and how they were able to stay focused in sport, school, with friends? Encourage them to share ideas or strategies that have worked for them in the past.

Developing Focus (15 Minutes)

Focus is a skill that can be developed over time. With practice anyone can train themselves to increase their focus. One practice activity is the use of a focus grid found at the end of this session. When doing this activity make sure that each youth has three or four different colored pencils, crayons, or markers. Tell the group they have a given amount of time to complete the following exercises. Start the timer after providing directions to follow during this exercise.

Focus examples:
- Start at 1 and count up by 3s
- Start at 54 and find the numbers going down towards 1
- Circle all the prime numers — the first few prime numbers are 2, 3, 5, 7, 11, 13, 17, 19, 23, and 29.
- Start at 19 and circle the consecutive numbers by 1s

You can change the length of time you allow for each one (many people find it difficult to focus knowing they only have 20 seconds to complete a task). For the final stage, add in a distraction (banging on a table, yelling, humming, etc.).

Focus to Win (10 Minutes)

Have everyone stand in a circle, and pick one person to go in the middle. That person can go up to anyone on the outside of the circle and say, "Darling, I love you, won't you please, please smile?" The person in the middle tries to focus on getting people to smile or laugh, while the receiver focuses on keeping a straight face. If the person can respond by saying, "Darling, I love you, but I just can't smile," then the person in the middle has to move on to another person in the circle. The person in the middle can do anything, except touch the person, to make them smile. When someone smiles they go in the middle and repeat the exercise.

Debrief and Transfer (5 Minutes)

Once you have completed the activities it is recommended to have the group debrief their experiences with the activities and to talk about how they can transfer what they have learned to other domains in their lives. You may want to ask the following questions:

- How would you describe focus?
- How can you stay focused at school/work/when performing?
- What activities can you do to stay focused on your long-term goals outside of this program/session?

Focus Grid

98	49	76	66	27	11	32	94	74	51
57	25	79	50	55	59	23	3	31	4
7	72	70	15	62	65	45	46	44	40
90	67	69	26	89	28	53	16	73	54
24	68	39	96	63	71	60	77	64	78
41	19	20	30	14	43	81	61	8	85
86	10	75	13	88	0	34	84	21	58
37	6	99	2	36	33	42	17	22	82
56	1	29	9	95	5	92	91	52	35
83	47	87	18	93	48	38	97	12	80

Notes

Learning to Relax

Successful people are able to rise above crisis by relaxing no matter what the external situation. Their belief in themselves protects them against shattering. — Adapted from Maxwell Maltz

Why Relax? (5 Minutes)

Ask the youth or group to think of times when it is important to be relaxed. Some examples are before competition, before a test, before learning a new skill, after working hard at something, and when they are nervous, too excited, or scared.

Learning How to Relax (30 Minutes)

Help the youth recognize that there are multiple ways in which they can learn to relax by practicing all of the relaxation activities provided in this section. The rationale for having multiple ways of learning to relax is that some will work better than others. Encourage the youth to try them all and choose the ones they think will work best for them.

Learning to Breathe

Ask everyone to get into a comfortable position, then close their eyes. Tell them that they are going to take three deep breaths when you say "go." Tell them that it is important that when they breathe in it should be slow and deep. They should feel it in their diaphragm (point out where their diaphragm is located). Have them take three deep breaths.

Muscle Relaxation I

Ask the youth to think about what a bowl of cooked spaghetti is like. Ask them to describe it. Tell them that when they are relaxed they might feel like a bowl of spaghetti. Ask them to get into a comfortable position, close their eyes and stay quiet. Once they are quiet ask them to imagine that they are like the bowl of spaghetti they were just thinking about. Remind them that their shoulders should be relaxed and their arms relaxed at their sides and they should feel like they could flop over like a piece of spaghetti.

Muscle Relaxation II

Youth can also benefit from progressive muscle relaxation, which involves tensing and releasing various muscle groups throughout the body. Use the following script to help youth develop this skill you can use an online recording (see Textbox 11.1).

Settle back as comfortably as you can and close your eyes. Start by taking in a few deep breaths. Focus on your breathing. That is the only thing you need to think about. Everything else you're worried about or have to do today will still be waiting for you when we're done.

First, focus on your left hand and forearm. With your thumbs on the outside, make a fist with your hand. At the same time, twist your arm gently to create tension in your forearm. Notice the tension in your hand and forearm. Focus in on this sensation of tension you are creating in your hand and forearm. Now, all at once, relax your left hand and forearm. Let the tension flow out. Notice the difference between the sensation of relaxation you feel in your arm right now and the sensation of tension that you created just moments ago. Focus on this difference (20-second pause). Now, take in a deep breath (10-second pause). Continue to focus on your breathing.

Now, focus on the left upper arm area. Push your elbows back into your chair until you feel tension in your upper arms. Don't push enough to cause pain, but just enough to cause tension. Focus in on the tension in your upper arms. Now, all at once, let the tension out and relax. Notice the difference in the sensation of relaxation you feel now and the sensation of tension you created just moments ago. Focus on this difference (20-second pause). Take in a deep breath (10-second pause). Notice how relaxed your left arm and hand feel right now. (When you have finished, repeat the procedure on the right hand and arm).

Now, for the muscles of the face. This is an area that has a lot of tension related to stress. There are three groups of facial muscles. To work on the forehead area, keep your eyes closed and raise your eyebrows up as high as you can. Feel that band of tension across your forehead. Focus on that tension, the tension that stress can create. Now, all at once, relax your eyebrows. Notice the difference between the sensation of relaxation you feel in your forehead now and the sensation of tension you had created just moments ago. Focus on that difference (10-second pause). To tense and relax the eyes and nose area, squint your eyes inward while crinkling up and pulling up your nose toward your eyes. Focus on the tension around your eyes and nose. Feel that tension. Now, all at once, relax your face. Notice the difference between the sensation of relaxation this area feels now and the sensation of tension you had created in it a moment ago. Focus on that difference (10-second pause). For the jaw area, while biting down on the teeth in the back of your mouth try to pull the corners of your mouth down into an exaggerated clown frown. Focus on the tension you are creating. Now, all at once, let your face relax.

Notice the difference between the sensation of relaxation your face feels now and the sensations of tension you have been creating just moments ago. Focus on this difference (20-second pause). Take in a few deep breaths (10-second pause).

Now, focus on the shoulders and neck. This area experiences a lot of stress. Pull your chin down into your Adam's apple until it almost touches your chest. Feel the tension you are creating in your neck. Focus on this tension. Now, all at once, relax your neck, and let it loose. Notice the difference between the sensation of relaxation you feel now and the sensation of tension you created just moments ago. Focus on this difference (20-second pause). Now take in a deep breath (10-second pause).

Now, focus on the mid-body area. While taking in a slow breath, draw your shoulders back and try to make your shoulder blades touch. Arch your back. Hold this position until you have to exhale and then exhale slowly, letting the tension flow out as you relax. Notice the difference between the sensation of relaxation you feel now and the sensation of tension you had created in this area just moments ago. Focus on that difference (20-second pause). Take in a deep breath (10-second pause). Take in another deep breath (10-second pause).

Finally, focus on the legs. Starting with the left leg, raise it in front of you. Now, point your toes toward the floor while keeping your leg out in front of you. Feel the tension you are creating in your leg. Focus on this tension. Now, relax your leg and let it fall to the floor. Focus on the sensation of relaxation (10-second pause). Now, pull your leg back up and hold it in front of you again. Point your toes back toward you and the ceiling. Feel the sensation of tension that you are creating. Now, relax your leg and let it fall to the floor. Notice the difference between the sensation of relaxation you feel in your leg now and the sensation of tension you had created in it just moments ago. Focus on this difference (20-second pause). Take in a deep breath (10-second pause). (When you have finished, repeat the procedure on the right leg).

Keep your eyes closed and focus on how your muscles feel right now. If you detect any tension, try to concentrate on and relax that area (30-second pause). Eventually, with practice, when you feel tension you should be able to send messages to this area to relax and loosen. Continue your deep breathing and allow yourself to become reoriented to the room, and then take two deep breaths and open your eyes.

Textbox 11.1 Relaxation Videos

Complete Muscle Relaxation Fun for Kids! (& adults too!)
- https://www.youtube.com/watch?v=aaTDNYjk-Gw

Progressive Muscle Relaxation for Children
- https://www.youtube.com/watch?v=UPQak4vxoRE

Debrief and Transfer (5 Minutes)

Once you have completed the activities it is recommended to have the group debrief their experiences with the activities and to talk about how they can transfer what they have learned to other domains in their lives. You may want to ask the following questions:

- Is learning to relax easy or difficult?
- When do you need to be able to relax outside of this program/session?
- What strategies or skills can you use to relax at school, work, family, or with friends?
- Are there some strategies you think would work better in different places?

Managing Emotions

The purpose of anger is to let us know that something in our life needs changing and to provide the energy to make a change. To get rid of anger you can change the situation or change how you think about the situation. — Garrison Wynn

How to Perform and Play Smart (5 Minutes)

To perform you need to learn how to control yourself so you can be the best that you can be. Have the youth or group think of examples when we may not manage our emotions very well. If the group is having trouble, give some of the examples below.

- Sometimes when we perform badly
- Sometimes when we are not allowed to do something we want to do (e.g., talk in class, stay out later, buy something at a store but parents say no)
- When you cannot figure out a problem or situation
- When you are faced with something that is scary or frightening

Explain that there are times we get upset with ourselves, but being upset does not help. Instead it is helpful to calm ourselves down, refrain from blaming others, and focus on what you did and how to correct it. There are four Rs to help you play smart.

Four Steps to Performing and Playing Smart (15 Minutes)

There are four Rs to help you play smart.

1. Replay – know what happened and what you did
2. Relax – take a deep breath
3. Redo – tell yourself what you need to do next time; make a plan
4. Ready – keep the focus on what you need to do next

Discuss with the participants that these four steps can all be done within five seconds and can usually be done in the midst of competition or a performance (e.g., prior to shooting free throws in a basketball game or during a tense moment of a performance). Once you have reviewed the four steps complete the Playing Smart Worksheet at the end of this session.

Having Everyone Play It Smart (15 Minutes)

This group activity is designed to encourage the youth to work together to come up with ways to manage their emotions. If you are working one-on-one with a youth it is suggested that you present each scenario and have them work through the four Rs for each one. Ask the youth to think of a scene or event that may occur in school, sports, with friends, or at home that may cause individuals to get upset and describe that scene. Some examples are listed below if the youth are having difficulty.

- You receive a test back from your teacher that you were sure you did well. She hands you a paper with a failing grade and asks to see you after class.
- Your parents ground you for breaking curfew last night. You knew you should have been home those five minutes earlier, but the decision is made and now you have to miss the school dance Friday night.
- You shoot the basketball too hard off the backboard and a player from the other team gets the rebound and passes to a teammate to start a fast break for an easy layup.

Have the group complete the following activity for the example you just described to them.

Replay–Imagine what just happened (the scene) and get one or two volunteers to describe it in their own words.

Relax–Think of ways to relax when in this type of situation.

Redo–Discuss what they should do in order to be ready for the next time the situation arises. Then have them imagine themselves redoing their plan.

Ready–Imagine themselves getting refocused and back into the game or performance ready to excel.

Debrief and Transfer (5 Minutes)

Once you have completed the activities it is recommended to have the group debrief their experiences with the activities and to talk about how they can transfer what they have learned to other domains in their lives. You may want to ask the following questions:

- What have you learned today about managing your own emotions?
- In what types of situations outside of this program/session do you think you need to work on managing your emotions?
- How can you use the four Rs in those situations?

Playing Smart Worksheet

Think of a time when you made a mistake and became upset. Complete this worksheet and share this experience with the group. Make sure that you use an example that can be done quickly.

Replay – Think about and write down what happened. Share with the group what happened.

_____

_____

_____

_____

Relax – Write down three ways you can relax. Tell the group the three ways you thought of relaxing.

_____

_____

_____

_____

Redo – Write down what you are going to do next time and imagine yourself redoing your plan. Share this with the group.

_____

_____

_____

_____

Ready – Refocus and get back into the game or performance ready to excel. Share with the group how you would do this.

_____

_____

_____

_____

Notes

Defining and Accepting Responsibility

"I must do something" always solves more problems than "something must be done."
— *Unknown*

Defining Responsibility (5 Minutes)

Ask the youth or group of youth, "What do you think responsibility means? What sort of responsibilities do you have in your life?" Use the following story if the group needs help answering the question.

As you get older, you are required to take on more responsibility in your life. Recognizing the fact that you are 100% responsible for your life is the starting point for all great achievement. Once you fully accept responsibility you will realize that no one else can live your life for you. Therefore, if you want something done, you must do it yourself. While other people may help you in achieving your goals, you realize that it is ultimately up to you to achieve them.

The key message is that when you accept responsibility you gain control, yet taking responsibility means accepting both good and bad outcomes of a situation.

Pointing Fingers (15 Minutes)

Label three different sheets of paper on different sides of the room, that say: "My responsibility; my fault," another "Someone else's responsibility; someone else's fault," and the third "Pure luck; pure chance." Make sure the papers are far enough apart for the youth to be able to move between those areas.

Explain that you will name situations and the youth are to run to the paper that best describes the probable cause of the event. Name both positive and negative situations (see the following examples), giving them time to move around. If you are working one-on-one with a youth, you place three sheets of paper in front of them (each one labeled as previously instructed). As you go through the examples, write each one on the paper in which they believe it belongs.

Examples:

- You earn an A in history.
- You're not invited to a party.
- You run for student council and you don't win.
- Someone steals your bike.
- You get caught drinking alcohol or using drugs underage.
- You win the lead in the school play.
- You earn a scholarship.
- Your boyfriend/girlfriend breaks up with you.
- You study hard, but you fail a test.

After going through this activity discuss with the youth the idea behind the examples from each scenario. The point you want to reinforce is that it is important to take responsibility and correct our behavior when things go wrong because of our choices, and also to see that bad things can happen to us that aren't our fault. When we fail, we need to realize that we all make mistakes and we're all learning. When bad things happen that are beyond our control, we need to recognize that we're in a difficult situation, but that we are not at fault.

Taking on My Responsibilities (15 Minutes)

Explain to the group that it is important to accept and take responsibility in all areas of your life. To help them recognize how they can do this, ask them to work on Taking on My Responsibility at the end of this session.

Debrief and Transfer (5 Minutes)

Once you have completed the activities it is recommended to have the group debrief their experiences with the activities and to talk about how they can transfer what they have learned to other domains in their lives. You may want to ask the following questions:

- What have you learned today about responsibility?
- What is one thing you can do to take on more responsibility outside of this session?
- How can you help others become more responsible?

Taking on My Responsibility

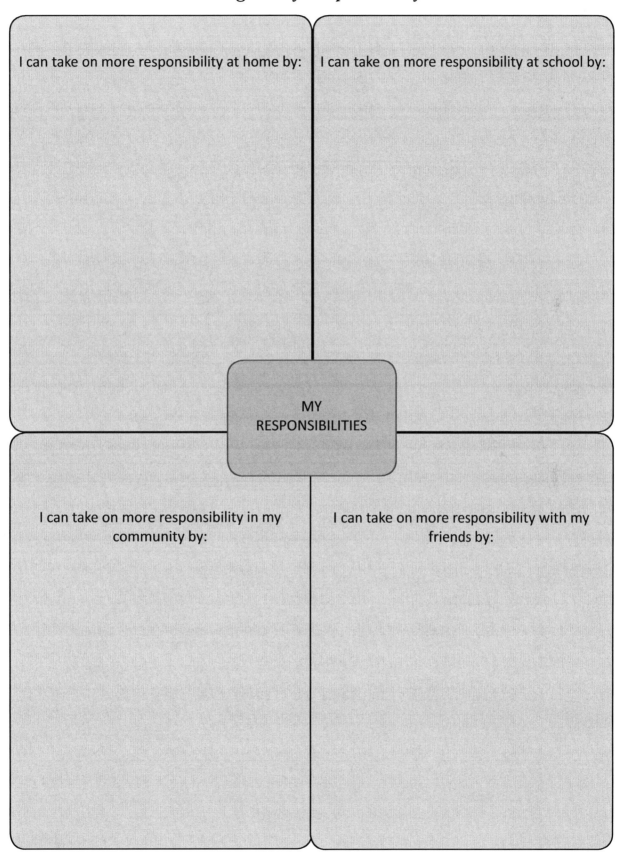

I can take on more responsibility at home by:

I can take on more responsibility at school by:

MY
RESPONSIBILITIES

I can take on more responsibility in my community by:

I can take on more responsibility with my friends by:

Notes

Respecting Others

"To be one, to be united is a great thing. But to respect the right to be different is maybe even greater." — Bono

What Is Respect (15 Minutes)

Respect includes taking someone's feelings, needs, thoughts, ideas, wishes, and preferences into consideration. It also includes acknowledging them, listening to them, being truthful with them, and accepting their individuality.

Respect can be shown through behavior and it can be felt. We can act in ways that are considered respectful, yet we can also feel respect for someone and feel respected by someone. It is important to feel respect for others because when the feeling is there, the behavior will naturally follow.

Ask the youth to think of someone they truly respect in their life. If working one-on-one, ask them to share that person with you. If working with a group, ask if some are willing to share and why. Once a few good examples have been shared, ask the youth to complete the Respect Worksheet at the end of this session.

Respect Balloon (20 Minutes)

Remind the youth or group that respecting someone means respecting their feelings, ideas, and needs. Here are ways to show respect for someone's feelings:

- Asking them how they feel
- Understanding their feelings
- Seeking understanding of their feelings
- Taking their feelings into consideration

Then ask the group what are some of the things we need to keep in mind as we learn to treat individuals fairly and with respect (e.g., Always ask yourself, "How would you feel if ..." before you are about to say something negative or rude to an individual).

Next, give everyone in the group a balloon. Have them blow it up and label their balloon with something that, to them, represents fair and respectful treatment. If working one-on-one with a youth, ask them to write all of the different ways or actions that represent fair and respectful treatment. Once everyone has a balloon, allow the youth to share what they have written and then discuss using the following questions:

- Is it difficult to act in this way?
- What makes it difficult?
- Why do you think some people don't do that?
- Do some of your peers disrespect or bully each other?
- How does disrespecting or bullying make others feel?
- What can you do to stop others from being disrespected or bullied?

As the youth or group proceed through the activity, remind them that this is what they want to practice.

Debrief and Transfer (5 Minutes)

Once you have completed the activities it is recommended to have the group debrief their experiences with the activities and to talk about how they can transfer what they have learned to other domains in their lives. You may want to ask the following questions:

- What have you learned today about respecting others?
- Outside of this program, who in your life do you feel deserves more respect than you give them?
- How can you show them more respect?
- How can you help others (e.g., family, friends) be more respectful?

Respect Worksheet

Think of someone you truly respect in your life. Write this person's name down as well as four points on why you truly respect them.

_____

_____

_____

_____

_____

_____

_____

_____

Notes

Managing Your Time

Time Wasters and Time Masters (5 Minutes)

To help the youth think about time management, ask them to make a list of the top five ways they waste their time throughout a day. If they need help coming up with examples, share some of the following ways.

- Facebook
- TV
- Daydreaming
- Playing video games
- Social media
- Texting

Then ask the youth to discuss how these prevent them from getting things done and how that makes them feel (e.g., more stressed, lazy, lethargic, unmotivated).

Where Does All My Time Go? (15 Minutes)

Explain or ask the youth whether it seems like there are not enough hours in the week to get everything done. Then explain that it may be true that they have too much to do and not enough time, or that it may be because they are not using their time as efficiently as possible. To help them gain awareness of their own time management skills, ask the youth to complete the Where Does My Time Go Worksheet at the end of this session. The overall purpose of this activity is to help youth gain more awareness on how much time things take and how they typically use their time.

Time Management Matrix (15 Minutes)

Explain that the time management matrix can help them develop a schedule that allows them to do what they need to get done (time master activities) and when they have extra time what they can do to have fun (typical time wasters).

Typically when we manage our time we can accomplish our goals and have fun too, but if we allow ourselves to be distracted we feel worse and less energetic to do what we need to do. There are three steps to improving time management:

1. Create a schedule with different time frames (e.g., a monthly schedule, weekly schedule, and daily schedule).
2. Evaluate the schedule, meaning assess what has been done and what may lag behind on an ongoing basis.
3. Adjust the schedule as needed (daily adjustments or long-term adjustments) based on your evaluation.

Debrief and Transfer (5 Minutes)

Once you have completed the activities it is recommended to have the group debrief their experiences with the activities and to talk about how they can transfer what they have learned to other domains in their lives. You may want to ask the following questions:

- What have you learned today about time management?
- Is there a particular area of your life in which you feel you could better manage your time?
- How can you develop a schedule for the different parts of your life? How can you combine these into one master schedule and time management plan?

Where Does My Time Go Worksheet

To assess where your time goes, complete the inventory below. Be as honest with your-self as possible. Some of the items are done every day, so those should be multiplied by seven to arrive at a weekly total. One item may be done any number of times a week, so you will need to multiply that item by the number of times each week you do it. After you have responded to all the questions, you will have an opportunity to see how many hours remain during the week for studying. Remember that there are 168 hours in a week.

Daily Activities	Example	Total Time
On average, how many hours do you sleep in each 24-hour period, including any naps?	X 7	
On average, how many hours a day do you engage in getting ready (shower, hair, make-up, etc.)?	X 7	
On average, how many hours a day do you spend eating, including any preparation and/or clean-up time?	X 7	
On average, how much time do you spend getting to and from school? Include the amount of time it takes to walk or ride the bus.	X 5	
On average, how many hours do you spend doing homework each day?		
On average, how many hours per week do you spend with friends (hanging out, parties, etc.)?		
On average, how many hours do you spend each week doing extracurricular activities (teams or clubs, music lessons, working out, church, etc.)?		
On average, how many hours a week do you work or volunteer?		
How many hours do you spend in class each week?		
On average, how many hours per week do you spend consuming media (watching TV, playing video games, being on a computer, or talking on the phone)?		

Time Management Matrix

Putting first things first means doing the most important things in life before doing things that are not as important. It means being clear about your priorities and acting on them. Categorize your daily activities, goals, and commitments into the four quadrants of the matrix. From urgent to non-urgent and important to non-important, you can begin to manage your time and prioritize your activities.

Urgent and Important (things you must do - priorities)	Important but Not Urgent (things that need to be done later)
Urgent but Not Important (things that distract you)	Neither Urgent nor Important (things that are not a priority)

Becoming a Leader

Example is leadership. — Albert Schweitzer

What Is a Leader? (15 Minutes)

This first activity is designed to encourage the youth think about what types of qualities they think a leader possesses. The activity can be done one-on-one or in a group setting. If working one-on-one, ask the youth to write down all of the qualities that a leader possesses. If working with a group, divide the youth into three groups. Provide each group with chart paper and have them brainstorm qualities that a leader possesses. After 5–6 minutes, bring the group back together and share the qualities each group came up with.

Ask the youth/group what they think the most important quality a leader should possess and why. Ask them, "When you think of the word leader, who does it remind you of?"

The Leader in You (20 Minutes)

Have the youth complete the Leader in Me Worksheet at the end of this session. The purpose of the activity is for everyone to identify at least five of the traits provided during the brainstorming session that they believe they have or want to develop to help them improve as a leader in the future.

Once the youth have completed the worksheet, ask the group to share one of the traits they they possess and how they will use that trait to exemplify leadership in the next week. Try to have the youth be as specific as possible. For one-on-one sessions, you can have a much lengthier conversation and discuss all of the traits. For those traits that they believe they possess, you can ask how they can exemplify it next week, and for those they want to develop you can discuss what they can do to develop those traits.

Debrief and Transfer (5 Minutes)

Once you have completed the activities it is recommended to have the group debrief their experiences with the activities and to talk about how they can transfer what they have learned to other domains in their lives. You may want to ask the following questions:

- What have you learned today about leadership?
- How can you show leadership at school, home, with friends, and in sports?
- How can you help others develop their leadership skills?

Leader in Me Worksheet

Use the list the group developed in the brainstorming session and write down qualities that you think you possess that makes you a leader, as well as the traits you want to work on improving.

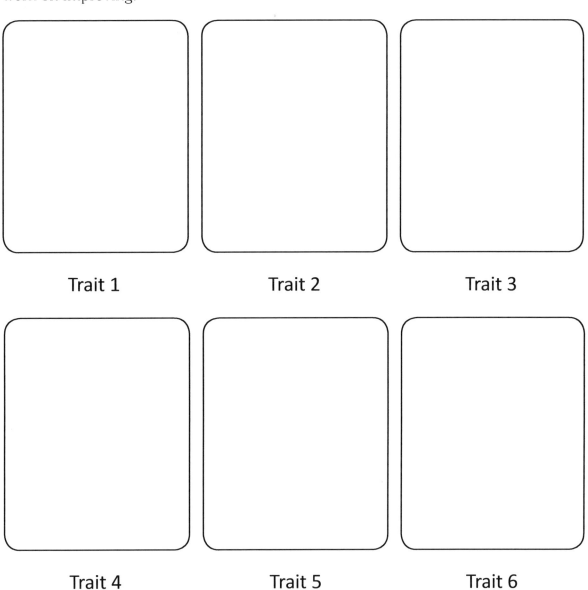

Trait 1   Trait 2   Trait 3

Trait 4   Trait 5   Trait 6

Notes

Developing a Healthy Lifestyle

One who has health, has hope; and one who has hope, has everything. — Arabian Proverb

What Is a Healthy Lifestyle (10 Minutes)

Explain to the youth or the group that participating in health-compromising behaviors can keep them from reaching their goals. Ask for a volunteer to name some health-compromising behaviors. If they need assistance, here are some examples:

- Smoking, taking drugs, or drinking alcohol
- Hanging around with the wrong people
- Getting into fights
- Breaking the law
- Dropping out of school
- Not being in good physical condition
- Lacking self-confidence
- Becoming pregnant or getting someone pregnant
- Not managing your emotions

It is important to convey that by avoiding unhealthy behaviors, it does not mean you are healthy. Ask the group the following questions: Sometimes when we think of being healthy, we decide that if we don't do any of the health-compromising actions we discussed, we will be healthy. Is that true? If so, why? If not, why not? What are some actions you believe are important to being healthy?

Ask the youth to identify healthy behaviors. If working one-on-one, you can list on a piece of paper any actions that they think are important to be healthy. If working with a group, share them out loud or divide into groups and have each group write down a list of healthy actions or behaviors. Remind them that some of the life skills they have already learned from you and this program can be examples of healthy actions or behaviors. Some actions or behaviors that are important to being healthy include the following:

- Getting enough sleep
- Smiling and laughing
- Being friendly
- Being physically active
- Eating healthy
- Setting goals
- Developing goal ladders
- Using the STAR approach
- Managing emotions by using the four Rs (replay, relax, redo, ready)
- Believing in yourself
- Creating a dream team
- Developing an action plan
- Learning communication skills

Discuss with the group why these behaviors are important to their health.

Committing to Health (20 Minutes)

Divide the group into three smaller groups. Have each group come up with a skit to demonstrate one of the health-enhancing behaviors they came up with in your discussion. Have each small group present their skit to the larger group. Watch the time to ensure each group gets a chance to present. If working one-on-one, have the youth identify three healthy behaviors they feel they are already doing well and then one or two they believe they could improve and discuss how the individual can work on doing this in the coming weeks or months. If you have time you can use the last session of this guide to help them develop goals for these new health behaviors.

Debrief and Transfer (5 Minutes)

Once you have completed the activities it is good to have the group debrief their experiences with the activities and to talk about how they can transfer what they have learned to other domains in their lives. You may want to ask the following questions:

- What have you learned today about healthy behaviors?
- What area of your life do you have to work on most to be healthier?
- How can you start engaging in healthier behaviors at school, at home, or in a sport?
- How can you help others develop healthier behaviors (e.g., parents, siblings, friends)?

Reviewing Goals and Personal Performance

Hold fast to your dreams
For if dreams die
Life is a broken-winged bird
That cannot fly.
— Langston Hughes

Review of Goal Setting (5 Minutes)

Remind the group about the initial sessions on goal setting and when we try to achieve outcomes we often are not successful because outcomes are not under our control. Sometimes we win or succeed even though we performed poorly. Sometimes we perform our absolute best but still lose or do not succeed. What we cannot control is how well our competition plays or who evaluates us.

One of the most important things to remember is the only element within your control is your personal performance. The best way to learn and improve is to compete against your own potential and previous best performances.

Developing Your Personal Performance (25 Minutes)

Each person in the group to imagine that they are getting ready to play a game or perform and that the competitor is their potential (which is defined as the best that you can be). Identify one skill that you want to improve to help you get closer to your potential. Then think about a goal they want to set to improve this skill.

Emphasize to the youth the importance of competing against yourself to better yourself. The goal can be related to school, home, work, friends, health—any area they want to improve themselves.

Finally, remind the youth of the four characteristics of a reachable goal: 1) important to you, 2) positive, 3) specific, and 4) under your control. Once you have reviewed these four characteristics, work on completing the My Personal Performance Improvement Goal Worksheet at the end of this session.

Debrief and Transfer (5 Minutes)

Once you have completed the activities it is recommended to have the group debrief their experiences with the activities and to talk about how they can transfer what they have learned to other domains in their lives. You may want to ask the following questions:

- What did you learn today about personal performance?
- What other personal performance/improvement goals do you have for school, home, or a sport that you can write down?
- How can you help someone else become their best personal self?

My Personal Performance Improvement Goal Worksheet

Set a goal and develop a goal ladder to improve a skill you know that will help you be better than you already are. Remember, this can be a skill that will help you improve in school, at home, with friends, in a sport or activity, or to increase your health.

My Goal

_____

_____

_____

_____

My Goal Ladder

Remember to develop a goal ladder. The first step is to identify the things that you need to do to reach your goal and then right them down in order (steps) so that you have a clear plan to achieving your goal. Write your goal here.

_____

_____

_____

_____

_____

_____

_____

_____

Target Date

Step 6: _____

_____

_____

Step 5: _____

_____

_____

Step 4: _____

_____

Step 3: _____

_____

_____

Step 2: _____

_____

_____

Step 1: _____

_____

_____

Conclusion

Y ou have now reached the end of guided activities for teaching life skills to youth. We hope you have discovered new ways of thinking about youth development as well as new ways in which you work with or mentor youth, individually or in a group, to help them become their best possible selves. It is through this work that we hope to help create contexts that help youth develop the skills they need to succeed. We encourage you to continue to use these activities and adapt them in ways that work best for your program or the youth with whom you work. In addition, we hope that this Guide has helped you gain more confidence in your work with youth and provided you with tips and tools to strengthen your programs as well as the relationships you have with youth. Finally, as mentioned at the beginning of the book, this is our attempt at "giving psychology away" and because we believe in social action, we hope that you will share your newly-gained knowledge and skills with others you know who work with and mentor youth. The more opportunities that youth are provided to develop and strengthen life skills the better prepared they are to take on life and to become contributing members to society. Remember Frankl's goal for his life--to help others find meaning in their lives. It is a worthy goal for you and for the adults and youth with whom you work. Imagine if every youth and adult found the meaning they wanted to have for their lives, and if they committed themselves to teach at least one other person how to develop meaning for his or her life. What a great world we would have! If that sounds as great to you as it does to us, remember—it starts with you.

References

Bloom, M. (2000). The uses of theory in primary prevention practice: Evolving thoughts on school and after-school activities as influences of social competence. In S. J. Danish & T. Gullotta (Eds.). *Developing competent youth and strong communities through after-school programming.* Washington, DC: CWLA Press.

Carnegie Corporation of New York (1989). *Turning Points: Preparing American youth for the 21st century.* Reports for the Carnegie Council on Adolescent Development. Wardolf, MD: Carnegie Cooperation.

Carnegie Corporation of New York (1995). *Great transitions: Preparing adolescents for a new century.* Reports for the Carnegie Council on Adolescent Development. Wardolf, MD: Carnegie Cooperation.

Pittman, K. (1996). Community, youth, development: Three goals in search of connection. *New designs for youth development, 12*(1), 4-8.

About the Authors

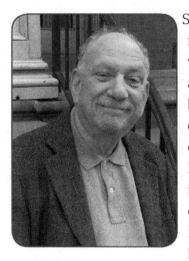

Steven J. Danish is president of Life Skills Associates and emeritus professor of psychology at Virginia Commonwealth University. He served as chair of the department of psychology and founder and director of the Life Skills Center. Previously, he held academic positions at Penn State University and Southern Illinois University following the receipt of his doctorate in counseling psychology from Michigan State University. Dr. Danish is a licensed psychologist and a diplomate in counseling psychology of the American Board of Professional Psychology, and a registered sport psychologist of the Sports Medicine Division of the United States Olympic Committee. He is a fellow of the American Psychological Association, the American Psychological Society, and the Association of Applied Sport Psychology (AASP) and is past president of the Society of Community Research and Action. In 2007, he was awarded the Lifetime Achievement Award for "Prevention" by the Society for Counseling Psychology. In 2008, he was awarded the Distinguished Alumni Award from the College of Education at Michigan State University. In 2013, he was identified as one of the top 21 psychology professors in Virginia by the StateStats.org. They noted that "he has earned praise from students, peers, and governmental agencies for his work helping veterans and their families cope with life after deployment."

He has written in the areas of military, counseling, community, sport, and life-span psychology; health and nutrition; and substance abuse prevention. He has received grants from the National Institute of Mental Health, National Cancer Institute (National Institutes of Health), the Office of Substance Abuse Prevention, the U.S. Department of Education, the U.S. Olympic Committee, U.S. Diving, and the Athletic Footwear Association.

In addition to his work as a psychologist, Dr. Danish has coached basketball at both the college and high school level and has consulted widely with professional and amateur athletes, allied health professionals, corporate managers, and police. He is a past member of the Virginia Governor's Commission on Sports and Physical Fitness, has served as the chair of the Virginia Tobacco Settlement Foundation Board, and presently serves on the Richmond Behavioral Health Authority.

He is the developer of the Going for the Goal (GOAL), SUPER (Sports United to Promote Education and Recreation), FREE 4 Vets (family, relationships, education and employment) and HELP 4 Families (health, empowerment, lifestyle and parenting) programs. GOAL is a winner of the Lela Rowland Prevention Award from the National Mental Health Association and has been honored by the U.S. Department of Health and Human Services. He served as part of the development team and curriculum coordinator of the life skills component for The First Tee, a national youth golf program, the NFL's Coaches

Academy, the Career Assistance Program for Athletes for the United States Olympic Committee, and the Youth Education through Sports Program for the NCAA. For the past decade he has focused on developing, implementing, and evaluating programs for veterans and their families.

He has been married to his wife for over 50 years. They have two sons and four grandchildren.

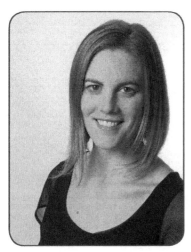 Dr. Tanya Forneris is currently Associate Director of the School of Health and Exercise Sciences at the University of British Columbia (Okanagan Campus) in Kelowna, BC, Canada. She obtained her Masters in sport psychology at the University of New Brunswick in Fredericton, New Brunswick, Canada and her PhD in counseling psychology from Virginia Commonwealth University. Tanya's expertise is in positive youth development and community programming. More specifically, the development, implementation, and evaluation of life skills based sport and physical activity programs to enhance youth development. In this work she has collaborated with local community, national, and international nonprofit organizations.

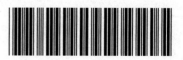